Brenda Lukeman (Ph.D., Adelphi University) has taught both psychology and philosophy. She has worked extensively with the terminally ill and run many training programs both in hospitals and in the community for those working with the ill and the bereaved. Her work arises out of her long-standing study of Zen. At the present time she is in private practice as a psychotherapist.

Embarkations

A Guide to Dealing
with Death and Parting

Brenda Lukeman

A SPECTRUM BOOK

Prentice-Hall, Inc., Englewood Cliffs, N.J. 07632

Library of Congress Cataloging in Publication Data

Lukeman, Brenda.
 Embarkations, a guide to dealing with death and
parting.

 "A Spectrum Book"
 Bibliography: p. 135
 Includes index.
 1. Death—Psychological aspects. 2. Bereavement—
Psychological aspects. 3. Loss (Psychology) I. Title.
BF789.D4L84   155.9'37   81-22743
ISBN 0-13-274522-4   AACR2
ISBN 0-13-274514-3 (pbk.)

10 9 8 7 6 5 4 3 2 1

ISBN 0-13-274514-3 {PBK.}

ISBN 0-13-274522-4

Editorial/production supervision by Suse L. Cioffi
Cover illustration by Jeannette Jacobs
Manufacturing buyer: Cathie Lenard

This Spectrum Book can be made available to businesses and organizations
at a special discount when ordered in large quantities.
For more information contact: Prentice-Hall, Inc., General Publishing Division,
Special Sales, Englewood Cliffs, NJ 07632

PRENTICE-HALL INTERNATIONAL, INC. *(London)*
PRENTICE-HALL OF AUSTRALIA PTY. LIMITED *(Sydney)*
PRENTICE-HALL OF CANADA, LTD. *(Toronto)*
PRENTICE-HALL OF INDIA PRIVATE LIMITED *(New Delhi)*
PRENTICE-HALL OF JAPAN, INC. *(Tokyo)*
PRENTICE-HALL OF SOUTHEAST ASIA PTE. LTD. *(Singapore)*
WHITEHALL BOOKS LIMITED *(Wellington, New Zealand)*

. . . for my Father.

This book is dedicated to my original teachers, Eido Roshi and Soen Roshi, and to my godmother, Tanao Sands.

Special thanks and acknowledgements go to my husband, children, and mother, whose constant love and support permitted me to complete this task. Particular thanks to Rabbi Ephraim Wolf, who invited me to join the minyans when my father died.

Contents

Foreword

Dying may rarely be easy, but perhaps it can be real. Friends, family, and professionals who are willing and able to stand close beside the dying have the chance now to be truly available to them, without limitations. Dr. Lukeman, through her own realness and sensitivity, has written a book that makes the process of working with the dying enriching and enlightening to everyone involved. *Embarkations* is a journey: first through the full spectrum of our own inner feelings and at the same time toward a full appreciation of the feelings of others.

This unique book is based on the premise that we cannot be of real help to another until we have access to our own emotions. The first half of *Embarkations* is a sensitive exploration of our feelings, needs, and fears when faced with death and parting. Dr. Lukeman provides practical processes and exercises throughout the book to help with this exploration. The exercises are derived from both traditional and contemporary modes of thought with particular emphasis on the contribution of Gestalt therapy and humanistic psychology. They are wonderful tools for introspection. As we become familiar with our own inner landscape, we see how this subject matter affects many aspects of our everyday life.

Embarkations is not a book to be read quickly but, rather, to be experienced and worked with personally and in depth. It is one of those books that has a profound and lasting meaning, with new depths appearing with each reading. *Embarkations* presents the perfect balance of deep philosophical and psychological concepts combined with the practicality of common sense. It is presented in a concrete, accessible, and very real way. It also provides the opportunity to see the meaning of love in our lives.

The second half of the book helps redefine and examine our relationships with others. It explores the true nature of communication, friendship, giving, and responsibility. Dr. Lukeman's purpose is obviously to bring light to a subject heretofore in darkness. Her approach is positive and at times even playful.

Embarkations is a vital resource for people in the health care community who are in contact with the dying, as well as any individual who is dealing with these issues in his or her personal life. Because everyone comes in contact with dying at some time or other, this book is a contribution to us all. Thank you, Brenda Lukeman.

Armand F. DiMele
Executive Director, The DiMele Center
    for Psychotherapy
New York City

Introduction

*There is a child within us to whom death is sort of a hobgoblin; him too
we must persuade not to be afraid when he is alone in the dark.*

Plato

This book is not about your death. It is about your life. Life and death
are occurring continuously, and yet we are not free to live fully until
we are finished with our fear of death. We are not free to love fully or
to extend a truly helping hand until we are able to let go of that which
we cherish the most. Living in the shadow, haunted by this un-
nameable fear, we may grow heavy, dull, and protected, losing the
precious life we want the most. Then death comes, and we are
shocked for a moment out of our stupor. We see that our life is not a
game and that our time may not be endless. We see that right *now* we
must say what has to be said and do what has to be done.

Time is like an arrow.

Many, many questions appear in our minds when someone close
to us is dying or when we ourselves are seriously ill. It takes a
while to realize that these questions do not have one answer. They
have many answers. They appear in many ways, in unexpected forms
and colors. They have different impacts on us at different times. In a

sense, a finger is being pointed in our direction. Questions are demanding a response from us. We cannot be free from answering them. Life itself is demanding an answer.

This book arises out of the deep need to find an answer, to make some kind of reply to the question of what happens when someone dies.

What has happened? One minute the person was here, talking to us, and now he or she is gone. We are confounded, bewildered, lost, and confused. Where has he or she gone? What happens to those who are left behind? There is no other time in life more painful; there is no other time when we feel more alone.

When someone we love dies, we die too. In our hearts there is no separation. And where are we, now that a part of ourselves has vanished? What happens in the long twilight passage that many of us must walk between the time of a severe illness and our death?

Usually we run from the pain of this matter into forgetfulness. When pain comes we offer drugs, we offer unconsciousness and denial. Instead of offering ourselves, we offer oblivion. We may not have ourselves to offer. Indeed, we are running away all the time only to avoid coming face to face with this matter, only to hide from our real selves.

But if only we stop running, even for a little, we can see that the only true comfort will come from understanding, the only true healing will come from the truth. If we learn to listen closely, we will find that the pain itself has a meaning. It's there to be listened to.

> *My friends, did you say you could not sleep last night,*
> *The heat of the summer bothered you?*
> *You could not find a cooler place.*
> *Why does death have to come to us?*
> *That question too, churned inside.*
> *Wait, wait until the evening sun*
> *Colors the mountain with its evening rays,*
> *You'll get more than coolness the moment when*
> *You answer that question, face to face.*[1]

Senzaki Roshi

[1]From *Namu dai Bosa: A Transmission of Zen Buddhism to America*, by Nyogen Senzaki, Soen Nakagawa, and Eido Shimano. The Bhaisajaguru Series. Copyright © 1967 by The Zen Studies Society, Inc. Reprinted with the permission of Theater Arts Books, 153 Waverly Place, New York, NY 10014.

This book is not written by an expert. There are no experts in this area. Only the dead can know the dead. Instead, it is written by someone who is simply willing to consider this matter and who has realized that this willingness is all. It's everything.

In this book you are also being asked for your willingness to stop running, and to look instead. Actually, this in itself is an act of tremendous courage; to consider these questions deeply even though you do not know where they are leading you.

There is so much fear about looking at death. We fear that if we face our dying, it will make us feel small and helpless. Actually, the opposite is true. In this way we grow alive and strong, reclaiming for our own the fullness of all our experience.

The entire book is constructed as a voyage, and each reader has his or her own particular journey to make. I appear as a fellow traveler, tossing questions and thoughts as if they were seeds into a garden. Some will grow and some will not. Each reader, each person, is a kind of garden, presenting a different kind of soil, a different condition of mind and heart, a different way of receiving the questions. This is especially wonderful. It is not necessary to relate to all the book. Certain parts will be especially for you.

Simply put, this is a book of seeds, and you are needed to participate and receive whatever you are able, to let your garden grow in whatever way it will. All the answers to the questions, all the kinds of flowers that can grow in the garden, already exist within you. Only patience and care are needed for them to appear.

This book is offered so that in the face of death we may become steady and simple and learn how to extend a truly helping hand.

Part One
THE INNER EXPERIENCE OF DEATH AND PARTING

chapter one
Facing Our Dying

A traveller—
let me be known thus
this autumnal evening.

Bassho

BEGINNING TO LEARN ABOUT OUR DYING

Our usual way of learning and knowing is based on the *scientific premise*. Here we are separate from the world. We take the world as being different from us, as our object, something to be conquered by our understanding. Here we observe, measure, and define in order to gain mastery and control. All our faith lies in our rational mind, and we feel that by thus molding the world, we are powerful, strong, and in command. Death teaches us otherwise.

We spend most of our lives searching outside ourselves for the things we already know. Running headlong to different disciplines such as psychology, theology, and sociology, we sense that someone else will be able to tell us the truth. We turn to priests, rabbis, and psychoanalysts. We think that by mastering a new vocabulary, we will have understood something more deeply. We consider that we are entirely blind—only in one sense is it so. There are many windows to view death through, but death is larger than all the windows. It cannot be classified or contained.

The path of science is not a bad path. It has its function and great usefulness, but it is not the whole story. There are places into which it cannot go. It cannot bring us ease at the deathbed of someone we love.

Where science ends, death begins. Death cannot be known through observation, as death has no form. We cannot gain mastery and control over death. When it comes time to die, nothing will stop it. We are never separate from our dying because we always carry it right inside.

In order to gain true assurance and understanding, we must simply enter a new realm of knowing. This is the realm of *intuitive knowing*. This simply means stopping our search outside and beginning to look and to trust within. This is the path of our own deep experience, a kind of pursuit that will lead us not to *know more* but to *be more*. Intuitive knowing does not talk to our brain but to our entire being. It is the kind of knowing that can show us how to walk calmly into the sick room and stay close beside our dying friend with wisdom, strength, and a real sense of beauty. It tells us that despite everything, all can be well.

In order to touch this possibility within ourselves it is necessary to ask a new kind of question, to view the events in our lives with different eyes. This book is dedicated to this new way of knowing. Throughout, there are questions, discussions and exercises, which will lead us to this different path. In this form of inquiry, we are simply directed to ask the *meaning* of what is happening to us. We do not try to mold or control our experience, nor do we try to *explain* it. Instead, we simply *meet with it*, become acquainted, and let it instruct us.

In one sense this is the path of humility. It requires the strength to let go of our need to control ourselves and our worlds. It requires the recognition that indeed we are not the most powerful, that there is something larger than us, and that we must simply learn how to connect with this in order to find our true source of wisdom.

Plato has said that we were born knowing everything, and that our lives simply consist of the process of forgetting. We have forgotten where we came from and where we are going. We have forgotten our purpose here on this beautiful earth. Now, looking within once again, we simply remember the knowledge which was always ours.

In the time of crisis, pain, and sadness, it is of the utmost urgency to learn how to reconnect with your own inner source of beauty and strength. This book is aimed at giving you the opportunity to see the workings of your own intuitive knowing. It is designed as a mirror for you to see into yourself.

> *Things are not what they seem, nor are they otherwise.*
>
> Buddhist Sutra

WHAT IS DEATH?

Death is the loss of our perception of the familiar world. We like to feel that we are at home, secure, and stable in the world. We aren't. We create many structures to give us a feeling of permanance and stability. Death takes them away, telling us that we are only transients here, that this is not our real home at all. Where is our true home?

When someone we love dies, we die. It is not only their death, it is our death that is happening, too. Suddenly, we are brought to the precipice, we may suddenly look into the vastness of space. We are thrown to the center, and then we return.

We may feel discomforted, restless, and sad. Our footing has slipped, and fear takes over, creating anger and dismay. Despite all our protesting, efforts, will, knowledge, and strength, there is nothing more we can do. We are left helpless and out of control. Death is simply reminding us that we are not in charge of the universe after all. There is something else we must answer to as well. Death is a tease. It forces us, despite our inertia, to look at the truth. An opportunity has happened to us.

> *When my aunt Sara died, I felt expanded, opened, sweeter, as though something lovely had happened to both of us. I left the hospital at about two in the morning and walked home alone in the city streets. A light snow was falling. I felt as though it were washing me.*
>
> *I felt confused. I just felt confused. Where was my father now?*
>
> *I still have Patty's stockings here and I keep wondering, where are her legs now? When we were little we used to run at the beach together. I still have her nail polish. All along I had a sister. Do I still have a sister now? Right now I am just uncertain.*

We may react by becoming humble, arrogant, or terrified. For a moment we may let go of our endless pretensions. More commonly, we start looking around for someone to blame. The doctors often become the villains. We need a reason and we crave to understand. There is a deep longing, often unconscious, to make sense of this event. Instead, we focus on trivial matters, blaming this one or that one for their insufficiencies. Tremendous guilt is created in others and borne in ourselves. This is a diversion only. We simply need to understand.

> *If only we had changed doctors this wouldn't have happened. He didn't do enough. I knew it all along, but I was afraid to take a stand against him. There was plenty we still could have done and we failed. It's as simple as that.*

This kind of feeling exists in so many that it bears examination. A feeling such as this grows into a gnawing guilt that persists for years. The deep sense of not having done enough, of not having been able to save a loved one leads many widows to dying within the year of their husband's death, or to major, unnecessary surgery. We do not feel we deserve to live while our beloved is dead. Guilt after death is just overwhelming.

In the case of a child dying in the family, spouses usually blame each other. All the times they did not love enough now appear in front of their eyes to be reckoned with.

> *I just couldn't look at my husband after Tommy was gone. I kept feeling he was blaming me. I kept feeling he was thinking if I had only been a better mother, more patient, more caring, this never would have happened. I kept wondering if he thought Tommy might have wanted to die. Neither of us could part with what was left of his bicycle. Even though the other children desperately needed our family to remain together, my husband and I separated that year. We just couldn't take it.*

This is such a common phenomenon that it needs to be dealt with. It cries out to be looked at and understood as a perfect example of our own lack of comprehension of death, of our misplaced sense of reponsibility. That which we can, and should be, responsible for we deny and overlook. In the places where we cannot really do anything,

we assume it is all our fault. This confusion must be slowly un-
ravelled so that our lives acquire balance and harmony. True responsibility can only come with seeing our place in the whole. It can
only be liberating, bringing fullness, clarity, and completion to all.

Unanswered questions creating this guilt and allowing this
bitterness haunt us heartlessly. If they go unattended, if they are not
heard, aired, and answered,it is their power that creates the persistent
pain.

Following are some of the questions you may have heard, or
may have needed to answer.

What did he do to deserve this? He was a good man.

She was so young. What about her children? Why her? It's too horrible.

*If it was me, I'd give him some pills. Why not? What is the value of
lingering in agony?*

*I saved and waited for my retirement. My wife and I made so many
plans. Just one year ago, I retired. Now this. Two months left to go. What
was it for? It was all for nothing. I feel as if I'm the victim of a horrible
joke.*

Intertwined within these questions are deeper questions such as,
"Why does death have to come to me? What does this say about the
meaning of my days? Someday I will die too. Where am I going and
where am I from? And why the suffering in between?"

Deep in the night, when the fear and the physical pain intensify
and it's so hard to sleep, these are the questions that are stirring.
What we are really dealing with here is the terrible anguish of
meaninglessness. It is the lack of knowing who we are and what our
place is in this world. It is the fear that our lives and the ways we have
spent them, may all have been some ridiculous joke.

*. . . I wept for my father too long and too much. I sat there weeping long
past when I should have. Then one day it struck me, I was crying for
myself too; crying because I was so damn foolish, with my life just
spinning in circles, always avoiding what I wanted the most. How could
a life like that make any sense in the face of dying?*

*It was still winter outside and little birds in the snow were
looking for food. I got up then, went to the window and looked out at*

them, searching for crumbs here and there. They were alive and my father wasn't. What about me? How alive was I?

Suddenly I felt jealous of the birds out there, free to fly from garden to garden. I felt happy for them too, and wanted to join them in the flight.

I got up then, went into the kitchen and took some bread from the pantry. Then I went out into the garden to give it to them. When they saw me, they didn't fly away, so I scattered the white crumbs on the snow.

Process

Use the following questions in the process of your own inquiry.

Look for just one moment into the past year of your life. What would you like to do over? What did you not do that you wanted to do? Write it down. Make it specific. Do not judge yourself. Just look at it calmly.

It may be as frightening to look at the quality of our living as it is to look at our death. Usually we avoid the matter, we run from it in whatever way possible through lies, facades, pretenses, and games.

Why is this matter so seldom handled? Let us begin to touch upon the fear that is gripping us. This fear has many aspects and is manifested in various forms. It is the deep fear not only of dying, but also of living, of living fully with freedom and truth. Fear of this nature may be considered the fundamental force that makes us turn toward security, boredom, depression, and other forms of lifelessness, rather than move boldly through our lives into new and unknown spaces. It is not death itself, but this fear which is so debilitating—a fear which holds us among the *living dead*, and brings us to the end of our days without a sense of fulfillment and meaning.

> *It is not the real death that is so frightening, it is the living death, the unlived life that haunts us.*[1]
>
> Henry Miller

Can we now find a way to move through this fear so that we may begin to live openly, perhaps not knowing what will happen moment

[1]From *The Wisdom of the Heart* by Henry Miller. Copyright 1941 by New Directions Publishing Corporation. Reprinted by permission of New Directions Publishing Corporation.

after moment? Is it possible to allow ourselves to be available to this much mystery and adventure?

Let us now begin to dislodge this fear. In order to do this, we will look at it, name it, trace it, and even make friends with it. We will start with some gentle exercises and processes. These processes are designed to help you know, experience, and dissolve your fears, thus opening new possibilities for your life.

Process

As you participate in these exercises, it may be valuable to realize that your responses are not very different from someone who is presently ill. By knowing yourself more deeply, you will feel less estranged from and more helpful to those who are dying and who need you.

This process may be done alone by writing down your answers. However, if possible, it is better to share your answers with a partner. When working with a partner, do the process aloud. First one partner completes the entire exercise (repeating the sentence ten times). The other partner simply listens, offers no comment and says "Thank you" each time the first partner completes the sentence. Then the roles are switched. Thus, each partner has a chance to complete each sentence ten times. When the entire process is over, the partners then discuss their feelings and responses to the material that came up for them. Both partners keep discussing their reactions to the process with each other until they both feel complete about. it. (These instructions apply to all the following processes of this type which are included in the text.)

Say whatever comes into your mind quickly in order to complete the following sentence. Repeat the sentence about ten times in a row, each time completing it spontaneously.

As I think about dying and saying good-bye:
1. *What I need right now to be a little less afraid is* _____
   Some Sample Responses
   a. "to hold someone's hand."
   b. "the sense that I can find some answers that feel good to me."
   c. "to be close to my children."

(The responses do not have to be clever or wise, just simply true. Let whatever wants to come out, come out. When nothing more comes, keep going anyway.)

2. *What I want from you right now, to help me be a little less afraid is*_____
   Some Sample Responses
   a. "to know that you won't think I'm silly."
   b. "for your eyes to look warm."
   c. "for you to hold me."

Now, if you are working with a partner, after the process is over see if you can give your partner whatever it is he or she needs. How does it feel now? Again, after the exercise is completed, share your feelings and responses about what went on. Talk it over until you both feel satisfied.

As we look more deeply into death, we are simultaneously looking into our own living. The fear a dying person is experiencing, the rage and loneliness, all arise from what he or she imagines it is like to be dead. The images we carry about death create our responses. But where do these images arise from? They can only come from our experience of life. Thus, our experience of death is still a *living experience*. It is the imagination of a person who is still alive.

This is such a crucial point, because once we hear that someone is dying, we write him or her off. To us, the person is gone long before he or she is really gone. We imagine the person is already dead, that his or her life and possibilities are over now and the agonizing process of withdrawal and abandonment begins to take place. It is crucial to see that this person is still very much alive. He or she is alive and presently experiencing the process of dying. The person is alive and now, more than ever, has great need of you.

It is even more crucial to see that you have great need of him or her too, and that sharing the experience of dying can greatly enrich and enhance your life.

I always believed that those who were dying were in some special place and that there was nothing more that we could share. I felt they were hanging between two worlds and that their dying was very different from my living.

Then my father died and I became obsessed with finding out where he was now. I felt he had gone to the land of the dead. Where was that land? Not knowing the direction, and thinking it was other than here, I began to visit the cancer wards and spend time with those who were presently dying to see if they had any better ideas. I soon discovered they did not. They were just as lost as I. They were just regular people who were now dying and in pain.

For some reason or other this astonished me. The more I looked at the faces of those dying, the more life kept staring me in the face. I might go to the cancer wards as long as I liked. Only live ones could answer my questions. All my answers and understanding, I suddenly discovered, could only come by turning around and looking at life. I was so stunned that I just knelt beside the bed of a lady who was tossing in pain. She reached out her hand to me and started to cry. Where had I imagined she was? I gave her my hand and we cried together while outside it started to rain.

Process

Let us now turn into our own lives and ask how we have experienced what it means to be dead. Where does our understanding come from? What are the images we are carrying inside?

Take all the time you need. Be gentle with yourself. Keep on remembering, there are no right or wrong answers. Whatever you see, whatever you feel is true for you, and it is fine. The art of these exercises lies in not judging yourself, not controlling or manipulating your answers, but in just allowing yourself to experience whatever response appears naturally. Do not be afraid of these exercises. Nothing bad can happen to you. If you begin to feel fear, just allow it to be there and then let it go. The less attention we give the fear, the less hold it has on us. Work with kindness toward each other. It is always helpful to have fresh flowers in the room. After you are finished, it is wonderful to have cookies and tea.

1. To be dead is _____
   Some Sample Responses
   a. "to be uncaring, not concerned with anyone around."
   b. "to be suffering. Only in pain from morning to night, then you feel like you're sinking."
   c. "to be away from my mother (father)."
   d. "to be alone all the time."
   e. "to be unable to say, 'I love you.' "
   f. "no pulse, heart beat, brain waves. It's very simple. No big deal."
   g. "... there is no such thing as death, as it's only some kind of dreaming and I'm not afraid."

Now, draw your answer. Write a short poem about it. Take a piece of clay and construct death. Share this with your partner.

2. To be alive is _____
   Some Sample Responses
   a. "to make love. That's it."
   b. "to be ready to give yourself completely."
   c. "to be involved and working hard."
   d. "to communicate freely."
   e. "to be close to your mother (father)."
   f. "to go dancing, peel potatoes, and not have to sleep so much."
   g. "to watch the flowers come up in the spring."

3. When were you most alive? Do you remember a time?
   Some Sample Responses
   a. "I am most alive when I help others. When I see I have done something to make someone feel better I have a strong feeling inside."
   b. "I feel most alive when it's morning."
   c. "In bed with a woman (man). The right woman (man). It's wonderful."
   d. "That's easy for me. When the whole family's together."

Look at the connection between living and dying. Always, in order for something new to be born, something has to end or die. Examine this within your own experience. What had to end before something new could appear?

4. The part of me that is most dead is _____
   Some Sample Responses
   a. "the part that's hiding."
   b. "the part that always makes excuses."
   c. "the part that stays stuck in the same rut year after year."
   d. "the part that's mean, tough, and angry often."
   e. "the part that doesn't want to try again."
   f. "the part that can't get up in the morning."
   g. "the part that asks the same question over and over."

5. The part of me that wants to be born is _____
   Some Sample Responses
   a. "the part that goes walking on the beach, even in winter."
   b. "the part that isn't afraid of saying good-bye."
   c. "the part that believes in him(her)self."

d. "the part that has curly hair."
e. "the part that forgets to be angry."
f. "the part that takes chances."
g. "the part that is fragrant."

The following is from the journal of Andrea, a seventeen-year-old girl dying of leukemia.

I didn't even know what it meant to be alive until they told me that I was going to die. At first it meant nothing to me, nothing at all. The word had only a strange, hard ringing to it. Something about platelets and corpuscles and my mother crying, holding the bedpost. She just stood there stunned, holding the bedpost, and my father's head was hanging. I just couldn't imagine not living, not being there with them anymore. It took a lot of days for me to wonder about what it meant then to be really alive, and how much I had lived in my seventeen years.

All of a sudden then, like a summer rainstorm, I wanted to live very much. I wanted to run on the streets and taste all the ice-cream cones, quickly before the summer ran out. I wanted to hug my mother and shake my father out of his stupor. Things I'd never thought of before. Things I'd have been afraid to do.

When we begin to see that death is approaching, time becomes new and precious. Time has always been precious, but we just never noticed it before. It is hard to waste time now. The question of how much time is left can become an obsession. Yet, it is necessary to clearly see that it is not the length of time necessarily, but the quality of our days.

With this realization comes the time to strip away the unessential, to come straight to the core of who we really are. Can we be brave enough to do this even if we have not in the past? No matter when we do this, even with only a few hours remaining, such an action will bring fulfillment and joy.

My mother's pain came from many sources, but mostly now I have grown to see, it came from her unfulfilled days, from the dreams she never dared make into reality, from all the things she did not do or say.

When your time runs out, there is no sedation at all for this kind of pain. There is no way to recapture what is gone, but the possibility for change exists every moment.

Process

This exercise has to do with guided meditation. It is best to do this process with a friend in the room. Let the friend guide you and read the instructions to you slowly, as you follow along with your eyes closed. It is helpful to play soft music in the background as the meditation goes along.

Close your eyes. Become as comfortable as you can. Imagine yourself on a road. The road is located in a beautiful place, somewhere that you have always loved to be.

Picture the road and the place carefully. You are walking slowly along the path. What kind of a day is it? Feel the air. Look around. Take your time.

Suddenly, up ahead, you see your death approaching.

Look at it. What does it look like? What is it doing? What does it want from you?

Speak to your death. Ask it where you are going. Ask it anything that may be important to you. Spend a little time in this conversation.

Now, you discover that you have about six months to live. You will not die now. Your death is fading.

Bring someone to you now, someone you want to be with. Who is it? Have the person sit beside you and talk to him or her. What do you want to say?

Remember the most meaningful thing about your life now. Share it with the person. Think of something you would like to correct or do over. Discuss that.

Now, think about the time you have remaining. How do you really want to spend that time? What is it you truly want to do?

Slowly, when you are ready, come back to the room. Feel the floor under your feet. Open your eyes. Give yourself whatever time you need to integrate the experience.

Now, share it with your friend.

Following is another excerpt from journal of Andrea.

Dear Mother,

... even as I'm dying, I'm living. I know you won't understand that. I know you will still think I'm strange, and now that I look thin and yellow if you look at me from outside, I probably look quite ugly to you.

But from inside, Mother, I feel beautiful. I feel bigger and bigger every moment, as if I'm going to burst out of this body and enter into another skin. Soon the whole universe will be my body. I'm living more, Mother, as I'm dying each day. I'm growing into something amazing. I wonder if you can understand that?

If you can, please tell me so.

chapter two
Beliefs About Dying

Coming from nowhere,
I ring the bell,
Going to nowhere,
I ring the bell.

Where am I from and where am I going? This is the basic question which is raised when we truly try to grasp our dying. Is this all there is, or am I headed for my ultimate home?

What exactly happens when we die? Biologically, the functions are ending. And then what? The question, "and then what"? is very, very crucial. The way in which we answer this question, either consciously or unconsciously, will determine not only our reaction to our death, but to our entire life.

Many belief systems have been created to explain dying. Whether we are aware of it or not, we are all run by these unconscious beliefs. We carry them silently deep within, often not even knowing that they are there. Then death comes and they erupt, causing us to tremble greatly. It is not death, however, which is making us tremble. It is the beliefs and images which we carry inside. In our fear and our grief, we are responding to what we feel is going on. These images we have of dying are often the same as those we have about living.

Is death terrifying, annihilating, punishing, awesome, beautiful, suffocating, releasing? Is it nothing? Is it magical?

Process

Let us look at our images about dying and living. Let us compare the two.

You may do the following exercise alone or with a partner. (If you do it with a partner, choose an A and a B. A should repeat the sentence several times and complete it spontaneously each time. B should just listen and respond by saying "thank you" each time. Reverse the roles once the process is finished.)

To me death is _____.
The truth about death for me is _____.
The truth about life for me is _____.
When I am dead I will be _____.
When I die I will feel _____.

Discuss the responses you had. Is death a condemning father (mother) for you? Is it a welcoming mother (father)? A friend? A monster? What would this imply for how you live your life?

Now, create your images of death. Draw them on paper. Mold them in clay. Look at them as if someone else made them. Now, change them, make them into images which you would like them to be. What would this imply for your living?

The images that we carry are an important part of the belief system that we have adopted and internalized.

A *belief system* is a group of meanings that we create. It is a way of interpreting and handling the endless phenomena which address us daily. There are different stages we go through in receiving and interacting with the world.

First is basic phenomena (the world out there; that which happens). Then, we have our perceptions of it. Next, we have our images, meanings, and expectations. Finally, we have the interpretation we ascribe to the event. This interpretation inevitably colors the way we perceive what is going on. We may not even ever perceive the phenomena directly, but just perceive our beliefs about it. This is a complicated and subtle matter. There are many, many ways of viewing and interpreting an event. The belief an individual holds will inevitably affect how he or she responds.

Most belief systems are unconscious. The more unconscious a belief system is, the stronger its hold upon our lives. We simply take a belief system for granted, as it becomes a basic assumption that we live by. Since it is never looked at or questioned, it feels like a fundamental reality.

A belief system is *not* a fundamental reality. It is simply a cluster of ideas *about* this reality. Reality itself is direct and immediate and needs no intermediary. No matter what we believe *about* reality, reality itself remains as it is. We can change our beliefs a thousand times, but we cannot change the basic phenomena. No matter what we choose to believe, someday we will all disappear. In order to know reality directly, we must put our beliefs aside.

Since the beginning of time, belief systems have been created around the phenomena of dying. Some say we are here only for a moment, a brief flash of light and then darkness. Others say we have come here for a purpose. Questions surround our belief systems.

What is our purpose?

Have we come to do penance? To wipe out bad karma?

Is this life a kind of purification?

Is it a school with thousands of lessons?

Is it good and necessary to experience pain? Will this pain wipe all my debts away?

When I leave is there someone I must answer to? (If there is, I may be terrified.)

Is there an accounting I will have to make? (If so, I'd better prepare for it.)

Am I here to help and give to others? (When am I going to begin?)

Am I here to learn how to be loving? (Is there a loving father or mother who will greet me wherever I am going? If so, I may be comforted.)

Will I come back many times, over and over? Is there plenty of time to take care of my business?

Since I have come, is it possible that I may have the power to stay here forever, (and simply be unaware of this possibility?) The Immortalists argue that this is so.

Is this life just a gift, a pleasure and blessing? Is it a wondrous dance for me to enjoy? Am I just here to experience beauty and harmony? (If so, there are lots of songs I will sing.)

How do you view your own coming and going? Until you come to real terms with this question, you may feel your life to be haphazard and aimless, floating from this thing to that. However, once this question has been looked into deeply, your life takes on a different aspect.

You may ask yourself, "How can I ever find the answer to such an enormous question?" But, of course, there is no one answer. Actually, the answer itself may be unimportant. It is the self-examination and questioning which really matters. This process of questioning itself will bring you where you need to go.

Death itself has no answer. It is not a question. Death itself is a koan.

A *koan* is a question given to a student by a Zen master. This question has no logical answer. It can never be solved by thinking about it. It cannot be known by searching. Yet, this question *must* be answered. It is not an incidental question. It is a matter of your very life.

Soon this koan begins to haunt you. It begins to ache inside. It wakes you up at night when you are sleeping. You don't want to answer it, but it won't leave you. There is nowhere you can run to hide from it.

You have no choice but to find the answer. You know that the Zen master is waiting. Even though you may grow to hate him, he will still wait patiently for you. Sooner or later you must bring the answer!

Someday you will see that you are the koan, and that this koan is your very life!

Until death becomes your true koan, you do not become really complete. Unimportant matters become blown out of all proportion. That which is precious is pushed aside. A koan restores everything to its proper order.

When your coming and going become your true koan, we become incapable of hate.

> *If we truly saw that death was immanent for all, could we be anything but kind, loving, full of compassion all the time?*
>
> Kierkegaard

The purpose of this chapter (and this book) is not to offer any ready-made answers, but to goad you into seeing the question. To begin to do this, we will look more deeply at what we truly feel about death itself, about who we are and where we are going.

Process

Here is a process to help you go within. This should be done with a partner, who is to read the instructions to you. (It can also be done in a group or a classroom. Some find it helpful to have soft music playing in the background as the instructions are read.)

Relax, and close your eyes. Become as comfortable as you can. Now, imagine yourself in a safe and lovely place. Choose a place where you would really want to be. See it clearly. Feel comfortable there.

Now, picture a road winding to where you are sitting. Along with this, see your death approaching. Look at it closely. What does it look like? Your death is telling you that it is time to die. Listen to these words spoken to you.

Now, you are being taken somewhere. Be aware; what is happening. See yourself die. How do you die? How does it feel? What is it like? Before you go, see the universe with you in it. Now, see the universe without you in it. Where are you now? What is it like? What are you now? (Take all the time you need to feel this through.) What do you need to make you most comfortable?

Now, visualize yourself ready to come back to life again. You can come back to any place and in any form that you would choose. Where would you come back to? See yourself there. What are you doing there? How do you look? Who would you be? (Again, take all the time you need to feel this through carefully.)

When you are ready, come back to the room here. Rub your arms and legs gently along the floor. Open your eyes.

Now, without talking, take some paper and crayons and draw a picture of what happened to you. Draw a picture of your dying. Draw another picture of who and where you were when you returned. Look at these pictures and see what they are saying to you. Share them with a partner.

Now, find a new song, your own song to sing about your experience. Or, write your own poem about this. Share what you are creating with another.

I saw you!
Your shadow after lunch.
Your little white shadow
slipping right through my
burning heart.
Where are you going?
I come? Yes, I want to
come! Just come?
Where are we going?
I know not how to
walk. I am ashamed
of crawling after you.
I know not!
I guard your wake and
sleep. I guard your day
and night. But it is you
who takes care of me.
I can offer only my body;
I will give it, so you can
sleep and wake.
You offer your being and
I am blind.
Tears of pain and joy
come to my blind eyes,
burning through my heart
on their way to you.

Where can we meet?
Let me settle into you, so
I can heal my burns,
I come.
Those few steps seem like
the path to eternity. I will
Make it—I have to heal.
The path is healing me, if
only I would not hurt myself
again and again.[1]

Swami Anand Vimalkirti
(written to Bhagwan Rajneesh just before dying)

From out of the deepest images and dreams that we hold, we create

[1]From *Zen: Zest, Zip, Zap and Zing* by Bhagwan Shree Rajneesh. Copyright 1981, Rajneesh Foundation, Poona, India.

our beliefs. These beliefs affect every moment of our living. Our understanding of our death and life are actually one.

Let us look now more directly at some of the beliefs that people carry.

> O Simmais, what are you saying? I do not regard my present situation as a misfortune. . . . I am no worse off now than at any other time in my life. I have as much of the spirit of prophecy in me as the swans. And they, when they perceive that they must die, having sung all their life long, do then sing more lustily than ever, rejoicing in the thought that they are about to go away to the god whose ministers they are.

> Plato
> (Socrates just before he dies to his student)

Some believe that we have a soul (which may pass through many lives). At death, this soul returns to its creator to be judged. After death we reap the fruits of our life here on earth. Our time on earth is a test and a trial. Perhaps we come here to be purified.

> The Rabbi of Ger once said, "Why is man afraid of dying? For does he not then go to his Father! What man fears is the moment he will survey from the other world everything he has experienced on this earth."[2]

> Martin Buber

Let us consider each of these different views seriously. Let us take each one in and hold it for a few moments. Taste it, know it, see what it would mean for your life if you accepted it into your being. Imagine yourself *really* believing the belief. Then picture yourself walking through your day. How would it be different from your day now?

> Someone asked the Rabbi of Ger: "Why do people always weep when they say the words in the prayer, 'man, his origin is of the dust and his end is in the dust'? If man sprang from gold and turned to dust, it would be proper to weep, but not if he returns whence he has come."
> The sage replied, "The origin of the world is dust, and man has been placed in it that he may raise the dust to spirit."[3]

> Martin Buber

[2]Excerpts from Martin Buber, *Between Man and Man,* Copyright © 1965 by Macmillan Publishing Co., Inc. Used by permission of Macmillan Publishing Co., Inc., and Routledge & Kegan Paul, Ltd.
[3]Buber, *Between Man and Man.*

What does the word *spirit* mean to you? Draw a picture of it.

> *Rabbi Zevi told this: "Some time after my father's death (The Bal Shem Tov), I saw him in the shape of a fiery mountain, which burst into countless sparks. I asked him, 'Why do you appear in the shape such as this?' "*
>
> *He answered, "in this shape I served God."*[4]

Martin Buber

Some feel we are here only to serve God, to redeem the world, and to make it beautiful. What could you do to make your world beautiful?

For others, death itself is truly nothing; blackness, loss annihilation. We enter the abyss and are simply destroyed. All beliefs are simply fictions, used to prop ourselves up.

> *And yet none of this priest's certainties was worth one strand of a woman's hair. Living as he did, like a corpse, he couldn't even be sure of being alive. It might look as if my hands were empty, but actually I was sure of myself, sure about everything, far surer than he, sure of my present life and of the death that was coming. Nothing, nothing had the least importance and I quite well knew why. From the dark horizon of my future a sort of slow, persistent breeze had been blowing toward me, all my life long, from the years that were to come. What difference could it make to me, the death of others or a mother's love?*[5]

Camus (from *The Stranger*)

In what ways are you as this stranger? Look and see. Odd as it may seem, we can encompass all of these points of view, at different times in our life. When we become conscious and aware of them, then we have the ability to choose which one we wish to live by. For some, there is an alternative to physical death. Physical death is not necessary.

> *Death is highly overrated.*[6]

Leonard Orr

[4]Buber, *Between Man and Man.*
[5]From *The Stranger* by Albert Camus, translated by Stuart Gilbert, copyright Alfred A. Knopf, Inc.
[6]From *Rebirthing in the New Age*, by Lenard Orr, Celestial Arts, Millbrae; Calf., 1977.

The idea that death is inevitable has killed more people than all other causes of death combined. Although we have been heavily programmed to believe otherwise, it is possible to go on living forever without dropping the physical body. Our unfortunate habit of affirming the power of death causes not only death, but also many illnesses and states of weakness leading up to death.

It is certain that there are people living on this earth who are more than two hundred years old, some much older than that.

All death is suicide. Your mind creates the death of your body. Your beliefs control your physical body. When you love your body as much as God loves your body, you can live forever.[7]

Leonard Orr

These Immortalists have devised a breathing therapy called *rebirthing*, in which they return to the time of their birth and release all negative thoughts, trauma, and memories, which lead them to believe that it is not safe and pleasurable to be alive. Then they fill their minds and bodies with thoughts of pleasure, health, well-being, and love. These are the students of Babaji.

For some, death is not a negativity. It is simply a passage into a larger state of being.

"Bhagwan, is there anything you can say about what is happening to Vimalkirti?" (A student who was dying)

"Nothing is happening to Vimalkirti, exactly nothing because nothing is nirvana. The West has no idea of the beauty of nothingness. Nothing sounds like emptiness—it is not so. Nothingness is not empty, on the contrary, it is just the opposite of emptiness. It is fullness, it is overflowingness.

One comes to a space where nothing is happening, where all happening has disappeared. The doing is gone, the doer is gone, the desire is gone, the goal is gone. One simply is, there is simply silence, but the silence is not empty, it is very full. The moment you are absolutely silent, absolutely attuned with nothingness, the whole descends in you, the beyond penetrates you."

Bhagwan Rajneesh[8]

"Be still and know that I am God."

Bible

[7]Orr, *Rebirthing in the New Age.*
[8]From *Zen: Zest, Zip, Zap and Zing,* by Bhagwanshree Rajneesh, Copyright 1981, Rajneesh Foundation, Poona, India.

Returning now to death as our true koan, our teacher, we go to the simple words of Suzuki Roshi and Soen Roshi.

Our life and death are the same thing. When we realize this fact, we have no fear of death anymore, or actual difficulty in our life.

I went to Yosemite National Park and I saw some waterfalls. And the water did not come down as one stream, but seemed to be separated into many tiny streams. So I thought it must be a very difficult experience for each drop of water to come down from the top of such a high mountain. It takes a long time, you know, for the water to finally reach the bottom of the fall. And it seems that our human life may be like this. We have many difficult experiences in our life. But at the same time, the water was not originally separated, it was one whole river. Only when it is separated does it have some difficulty in falling.

After we are separated by birth from this oneness, as the water falling from the waterfall is separated by the wind and rocks, then we have feeling and pain. When you do not realize that you are one with the river, with the universe, you have fear. Whether it is separated into drops or not, water is water. Our life and death are the same thing. When we realize this fact, we have no fear of death anymore, and we have no actual difficulty in our life.[9]

Suzuki Roshi

The sound of the gong
forever
in the spring dawn.[10]

Soen Roshi

[9]From *Zen Mind, Beginner's Mind,* by Suzuki Roshi, Weatherhill, 1970.
[10]From *Namu dai Bosa: A Transmission of Zen Buddhism to America,* by Nyogen Senzaki, Soen Nakagawa, and Eido Shimano. The Bhalsajaguru Series. Copyright © 1976 by the Zen Studies Society, Inc. Reprinted with the permission of Theater Arts Books, 153 Waverly Place, New York, NY 10014.

chapter three
Attachment and Loss

What do we have that we can lose?

We come into life empty-handed and then expect to grab and hold onto everything. Immediately we make claim for ownership. "This is my mother! She can't go away!"

Some enormous hunger begins to develop and grow. What exactly are we hungering for? First it is only food and love that we are demanding. In the beginning it is easy to find satisfaction, but soon this craving grows more subtle. Our so-called needs become more and more intricate. We want everything. We want to receive, to hold, to possess. We want to have everything and to have it forever.

A little child in the store with his or her mother does not know where to look first. The child grabs whatever he or she sees. The child's toys are his or her toys; his or her friends are his or her friends and the child insists that they may not go away! This kind of attitude is hard to outgrow. We feel we are the center of the universe and that everything exists for our pleasure. We fight for our portion and then protect what we have with our very life. When death comes it is seen as a villain which is taking our goodies away. But what do we own? In truth, what really belongs to us? Even our bodies have a life of their own.

The very process of our lives may be said to be a process of becoming hungry, searching for food, and then becoming hungry

26

again. But we must stop to absorb and digest, we must be willing to discard the waste. We take in many goodies, but what are we willing to return to the universe? Certainly not those that we love.

There are many kinds of foods that we begin to require as we grow; emotional food, intellectual food, social food, and spiritual food. The journey of our lives may be said to be the act of discovering the different kinds of food we need for our nourishment, how to take them, eat them, use them, digest and absorb them, and then how to let them go. We could not live very long if we did not go to the bathroom.

Nobody likes to talk about the bathroom. But it is very important if we are going to talk about death, about attachment and letting go. No one can live just eating forever. We must learn to be satisfied and to let go.

For many of us in this society, our lives are centered around accumulation; around eating and growing fat. We become very proud of what we have accumulated; money, degrees, skills, friends, information, property, lovers, walls of paintings and photographs. Soon we are full and overflowing. We are so full we can hardly move. Our houses are filled with possessions, and still we search for something more. It is not so easy to clean out the drawers. We have not yet learned the value of empty space. We may not have yet learned to make friends with our hunger and not let it be a devouring force.

Inevitably, along with the process of accumulation, the process of attachment appears. We become so afraid of losing that which we have accumulated. Everything seems precious, no matter what. There is little real discrimination. We hold onto everything for old time's sake. Why? Never mind. We do not have time to stop and ask, "Is this valuable? Is this meaningful? Do I need it, do I want it anymore?" Instead, our energy is spent on hunting for the perfect object, job, or relationship. We are driven to *do* more and more, have more and more, to feel that we are becoming bigger and better, wiser and finer. There is the overwhelming need to *become* something wonderful; to *do* something significant, to make our stay here meaningful.

We feel that we must earn our keep here and constantly prove that we are wonderful. We do not see that we are perfect already, beautiful already, that we were born whole and complete. Nothing extra needs to be added.

All I ever wanted, mother, was for you to know me, see me, and love me just as I was. I wanted to strip away all of the lies I had to tell you, all of the prizes I had to win. I wanted to stop running madly, living out your life for you. I wanted you to learn how to be happy, and I wanted to learn it, too.

Andrea, a seventeen-year-old girl dying of leukemia

stopping,
and counting every sound,
stopping,
and seeing every stone,
stopping,
and letting in the wind,
stopping,
and not having to be somebody

Peter Rosegarden, an eleven-year-old boy

. . . a student was searching for a teacher to show him the best way to live. After many weeks of travelling on the high mountain, he came to an old Zen master's hut. It was a simple hut, sparsely furnished and absolutely clean. The old teacher invited him in and asked him to have a cup of tea. The student waited patiently as the water boiled for the tea. Finally, when it was ready, the teacher prepared a fine cup of tea. The student held out his cup to receive it, and the teacher poured the tea. He continued to pour and pour even after the cup was full. Soon the hot tea spilled out over the edges, burning the student's hand. The student cried out in alarm. "Why are you pouring hot tea over the edges like that?"

"Just like this cup," the teacher replied, "you are filled to the brim with yourself, your thoughts, feelings, and opinions. If you want to learn something from me, first you must empty your cup. You must make room for something new to enter."

Old Zen story

Just like the teacher in the little hut, death comes to help us to empty ourselves. It does not mean to harm or to punish, but instead to stir our awareness, to push us a little out of the sleep we are having. We are simply being taught to loosen our grip.

Why do we attach and cling so tenaciously? What creates this kind of response? It seems so automatic, so natural and fundamental that we do not question it at all. Attachment *is* usual, but not natural. Certainly, it is not necessary. It arises only out of our deep confusion about who we truly are, where we are, and what is really going on. It arises out of misunderstandings about the nature of relationships. It comes out of fear, out of feeling abandoned. We may not yet see that we can never be abandoned. We feel the tighter we hold on, the less frightened we will be. The opposite is true. The gripping itself creates the fear.

Then one day death comes to show us that we are grabbing only at the wind. There is really nothing that we can hold onto, and the tighter we hold, the more we crush whatever it is in the palm of our hands. This sense of crushing and being crushed is at the very core of the pain we experience. It is our resistance to the flow of life.

> *Butterfly,*
> *Butterfly,*
> *You'll never catch me.*
>
> Eshin

> *"But I want my mommy to stay with me forever."*
> *"What is forever, Pamela?"*
> *"I don't know. I heard about it in a book somewhere."*
> *"What does forever look like, Pamela?"*
> *"(smiling a little) . . . maybe my freckles will last forever?"*
> *"Can you draw me a picture of forever?"*
> *"This is silly, but I'll draw it anyway."*
> *"And what happens when forever goes away?"*
>
> Pamela, a nine-year-old cancer patient

Process

It is very helpful to become clear and concrete about the concept of forever, which somehow walls us in. We have a strong sense of things lasting forever. But what is forever? It is only a figment of our imagination. Can we taste it? Touch it? How do we really know about forever? Once we begin to examine this closely the fearful aspects of the concept dissolve spontaneously.

What is forever? Look at this very specifically. Make a drawing, or shape it with clay. How do you interact with forever during your life, day by day?

Particularly during a time of illness and loss, we begin to search madly for something which is stable, which will not alter or go away. What is it that does not change or go away?

Examine this closely. Some will reply that God does not alter. God is eternal.

Then it is necessary to find God for ourselves, moment after moment in the middle of the flux. It is necessary to take the eternal with you directly back into the sickbed. How do you do this?

Just a concept is not enough. It does not bring ease when we are in great pain and close to dying. It is necessary to make this concept concrete, vivid, and thoroughly real.

Painted cakes do not satisfy hunger.

(Zen saying)

Process

If you want to find God, where do you look for him/her?

"He sleeps next to my mother's bed."

"In the rainbow."

"When it snows, I see God's face smiling."

"In chocolate chip ice-cream cones."

During a time of serious illness and death, many begin to think about God. Some feel ashamed and uncomfortable just to talk about it aloud. They feel that by now they should have outgrown such foolishness. Others carry a secret longing to feel God's presence with them.

It is enormously helpful to discuss this openly. It doesn't matter what one's different beliefs are, just to open this up for discussion relieves a great deal of the tension and stress.

Mrs. Adams: (laughing, slightly embarrassed) . . . well, of course I haven't talked, or really thought about God since I was a child. We outgrow that kind of thing. I did go to church occasionally, but well, I don't discuss it much. But yes, I must tell you, I have been wondering about it again. Recently all of this has been with me. It's nice of you to ask.

Often, all that is needed to open the area is to gently remark, "I sometimes think about God, do you?" It is then amazing to notice how a patient, friend, or relative will begin to pour out their thoughts, fears, and desires.

Now it is particularly important to be entirely open to the feelings of the other person and in no way to offer your own point of view. Your point of view is your own and not really relevant to the other person. At this time, it is most helpful to offer an open, present, accepting attitude so that you may create a situation in which the patient, friend, or relative is free to explore what is truly going on inside.

Just the freedom to be listened to, not judged, not taught, just really listened to, is tremendously healing in itself. A patient, friend, or relative will begin to feel as if some gift has been given to him or her.

> *Seeing the smile*
> *in your eyes,*
> *I have forgotten,*
> *that people die.*
>
> Old Zen saying

This search for God, for meaning, or for eternity is another form of the search for yourselves.

> *... Man senses in himself the loss of something valuable. He does not know where to begin to search for it. ...*
>
> *My ox, my ox,*
> *It has run away,*
>
> Old Zen saying

In this search for ourselves, for self-definition, and for self-understanding most of us become detoured by the static sense of identity, by the static sense of God. This is the sense that my world and I are stable and stationary. This is the sense that death never comes and that I will go on, in my present form, continuously. This is the nature of all delusion.

This kind of misunderstanding comes out of identifying with an object. I am my job, achievement, name, my relationship. This is how I know myself. I am this and not that. This group is good, the other is bad. There are boundaries; strangers and friends.

Like the object I identify with, I begin to feel static too. I become dependable, predictable, and unable to move or change. Somehow I do not identify myself with the basis of all life, that which is moving, changing, and in constant flux.

> Just simply alive,
> Both of us, I
> And the poppy.[1]
>
> Shiki

The poppy is alive and blowing in the wind, but my static sense of identity is based upon a world that is stable, secure, and does not change. It certainly does not blow in the wind.

But I do change. I lose my possessions. My wife goes away. My hair grows thinner. I try to pretend this isn't happening and try to keep everything the same. This very effort causes my suffering. I spend my life desperately trying to hold everything together and yet, no matter how much I try, everything constantly falls apart. But still I feel that my security and my identity can come only from holding everything in place and keeping myself intact.

Naturally this false sense of security is constantly being threatened. It has to be. It is based upon that which is not true. It can be, at best, only a holding action. Deep down I know it is not true. Then death comes and reminds me that I am floating in the wild ocean seated only in a cardboard boat.

"Is there a real ship somewhere I can board? Can I learn to become one with the ocean? Who am I anyway?"

Process

Right now, pick someone who is in the room with you, anyone, and give the person something that belongs to you. If you are alone, choose someone you know and write what you would give the other person on a piece of paper.

What are you willing to give away? What do you feel that you have to hold onto? Why? What do you want back from that person? What are you willing to ask for directly?

---

[1]From *Peonies Kana: Haiku by the Upasaka Shiki,* translated by Harold J. Isaacson. The Bhaisajaguru Series. Copyright © 1972 by Harold J. Isaacson. Used by permission of Theater Arts Books, 153 Waverley Place, New York, NY 10014.

What are you willing to give away?
"My handkerchief."
"Some money."
"I want to give you my seashell necklace because I feel you are suffering so much. This necklace has made me happy."
"A kiss."
"I'm afraid to give anything away."

What do you feel you have to hold onto?
"My pocketbook."
"Everything."
"My dreams."
"My mother or father."
"My self-respect."

What do you want back from that person?
"I want you to like me, to think I'm nice."
"I want you to hold my hand tightly."
"I want all your money."
"I want you to praise me."

What are you willing to ask for directly?
"You know, it is very, very hard to ask for anything."
"I can't bring myself to ask for love."
"If you have to ask for it, then it isn't worth anything."

It is excruciatingly difficult for those who are ill and dying to ask for their needs to be met directly. When we feel we have nothing to give in return, it is unbearable to take, to feel like a beggar.

Often the dying feel so useless, so empty, and so much of a burden. It is as though they had nothing to offer. Under these conditions, we can demand and harangue, but it is almost impossible to reach out truly and ask to receive. A deep sense of shame pervades the dying. In order to be able to receive joyously, we must always be aware of what it is we are offering in return. Through this kind of awareness, we develop a sense of our value.

How do you have your sense of value? What do you give to others?

For those in contact with the dying, here are some questions which are valuable to consider. What does this person give to you? What kind of lesson, gift, value, do you receive from being with the dying, or with the very ill?

First, you must find answers that are absolutely truthful for you, and then communicate your answers *directly* to the person. Tell the person what he or she is *giving* to you. You may even ask directly what the person feels he or she now has to offer. Discuss this openly.

A wonderful question to ask is, "What kind of gift do you want from me? Will you let me give it to you?"

> *Dried salmon*
> *received, and oranges*
> *given in return.*
>
> Shiki[2]

When, in an interaction, the giving only goes one way there is a block to healthy flow. Something destructive may be going on. When we find that we cannot give (or take) from another, then it is time to look at what it is we are really holding onto. It is usually tied up with our sense of identity, with our clinging and not letting go.

Process

Please answer the following questions. (You may answer these questions in a variety of ways: draw a picture, if you like, or write a poem, make a collage.)

What can I lose and still be me?
What can I acquire and still be me?
What kind of image of myself am I holding onto?
How do you wish others to see you?

What can I lose and still be me?
"My mother."
"My job."
"My teeth."
"Not my name. . . ."
"My old clothes."

[2]Isaacson, *Peonies Kana: Haiku by the Upasaka Shiki.*

What can I acquire and still be me?
"A car."
"A new house."
"Lots of flowers."
"A new boyfriend."

What kind of image of myself am I holding onto?
"I have to be perfect all the time."
"I'm beautiful."
"I'm generous."
"I'm kind."
"I'm successful in everything that I do."

> *I was not sick for one day before my retirement. Now, this is my second heart attack in a row. After I stopped working, I fell apart. I felt lost. I didn't know what to do with myself anymore. I felt like I had nothing to contribute to anyone.*
>
> James Traubin, a sixty-five-year-old retired executive

A very high percentage of men become ill and die shortly after their retirement. Here the sense of identity has been based upon the role they have assumed. Now that the role is gone, they are bewildered and disoriented.

> *I managed a big company for years. I was tough too. The men thought I was tough, some of them didn't like me. But I knew what I was doing. Now, look at me. I don't know anything anymore. And I'm scared. I'm really scared.*
>
> Frank Slayton, a sixty-six-year-old retired manager

The job, the role, the family are all props that we live with continuously. They are wonderful adjuncts to our existence, but we must see beneath their function to the very essence of who we truly are.

Many widows and widowers grow very ill and die within a year of their mate's death. In part, this is through identification with the mate. Again, the question arises, who am I now that he or she is gone?

The very quality and direction of our life is based upon our sense of who we are. The deeper this sense is rooted, the richer and fuller our lives become.

During the Great Depression, many jumped from windows. Suddenly, the money was gone. They *were* their money. Who am I when my money is gone? Nothing, no one, so they jumped.

The anguish of being nothing, of having nothing, is the most intense anguish of all. It is not the physical death that is the most painful, but the sense of not existing while living, of not being real, being no one, of having no being, the absolute despair of not being a person, not being worth anything at all.

How do we know that we are a person? Through what we have accomplished? Through our feelings? Through the loving eyes of another? Through knowing what we mean to them?

This is knowing ourselves from the outside in; wanting corroboration, affirmation, acknowledgment from the world outside. Our entire lives may be spent looking in the mirror of another's eyes. When another dies, it may then feel like it is our very own soul that they are taking into the darkness.

The basic assumption behind this is: Who am I if I don't mean something to someone? Through a relationship we seek our identity.

Process

Look at the ways in which you identify yourself. Think of a person you care for greatly. Picture yourself with that person now.

With _____ I am _____.

Without _____ I am _____.

Pick someone else and repeat this exercise. Notice how your sense of identity changes with the different people you choose.

Not knowing who we are, we cling to others. . . .

By being so dependent upon the other's perception of us, we are seeking our source and value from without rather than from within. Thus, we become always vulnerable to the other's moods and responses. Also, we are always vulnerable to the possibility that they will take their love away. This sense of vulnerability makes us cling even harder. The clinging, demanding, and sense of ownership is then wrongly mistaken for love.

... Dear Mother,

You feel you have a right to hold onto me this way, to ask of me, to demand everything. You feel we are bound by some invisible bond that I for one, never agreed to, welded by an unspeakable tie. I do not want to be welded to you. I do not want you to miss me. I do not like the look in your eyes. It is harder and harder for me to have to pretend and say that I love you. If you really loved me, you would leave me alone. Please do not bring me anymore candy.

Andrea, a seventeen-year-old girl dying of leukemia

This fear that the other will take their love away is especially activated when someone is dying. Often we feel that by the very act of dying, the other is rejecting us, purposely withdrawing his or her love.

There is so much sadness at the bedside of the dying, such a tremendous sense of loss and losing. And yet, what is really being lost? Who is being taken away? How often do we know so very little about the person we are losing? How much have we truly shared of ourselves? How much have we opened and touched deeply?

We say over and over how we love this person, and yet if this beloved starts to change in a way that is not to our liking, if they might want to leave the relationship, then our so-called love turns to torment and hate. We might even want to throw them away. This is love mistaken for possession.

What has this got to do with really loving another? This is only a mirage of love, a counterfeit coin. This is just a branch from the tree of attachment.

... if they come we welcome: if they go we do not pursue.

Old Zen saying

Real love makes no claims or demands, it gives the other freedom and space. Real love cannot be taken away. It does not *belong* to anyone. It is always present, always available, as plentiful as the air you are breathing.

In order to taste this real love, we need only to *let go* of that which we are holding onto. It is this very act of holding on that keeps all true nourishment from us.

All that we can hold onto is only temporary and has to change, depart, vanish. All that which is of true value is here forever. We cannot hold it and we cannot let it go.

> *three times it cried*
> *and was heard no more,*
> *the voice of the deer.*

> Old Zen saying

chapter four
Saying Good-Bye:
Grief and Mourning

The long night,
The sound of water,
Says what I think.[1]

Shiki

There is no death and there is no parting. Yet we meet, touch, and have to go. We suffer so much, feeling that our loved ones are leaving and that we are ultimately alone. Deep chords of abandonment resonate within. Watching this passage, we may become grievous and sad. Sometimes the grief is so overpowering, the fear of the night so enormous, that we cannot even bear to live and try to love again.

"How can I bear to love you if I know that you will go away?" Being with a loved one who is dying, we see only that which we are losing. We may not yet be able to see that which cannot be destroyed.

Fear can take over. We fear being close. We fear really touching, tasting, and knowing each other. This closeness can seem like the greatest danger. There are so many walls we erect for protection. But living behind our walls, we grow lonely and sad. We must develop enormous compassion for one another, living as we do, so walled in by fear.

[1]From *Peonies Kana: Haiku by the Upasaka Shiki,* translated by Harold J. Isaacson. The Bhaisajaguru Series. Copyright © 1972 by Harold J. Isaacson. Used by permission of Theater Art Books, 153 Waverly Place, New York, NY 10014.

... I was always really afraid of my father, afraid to know who he really was. I was afraid to share my true feelings with him, to let him know how very much I cared. Then one day, he was gone, and suddenly I began to feel all the love for him I had never expressed.

Maybe it was safer this way, easier to love him when he wasn't there. It's easier to love a memory than a real person in the flesh and blood.

Most of our lives may be said to be retreating from love, holding back, waiting for the perfect moment or perfect person, or waiting for the other person to give to you first. There is no perfect moment. This is the perfect moment. Every moment is the perfect moment, every person is the perfect person. It's simply a matter of whether or not you are willing to love—and to share it.

When our loved one is dying, it may seem too late to start sharing. We may not be used to talking to him or her. We may even be afraid of saying good-bye. But, until we can really say good-bye and be able to fully part from a person, we can never dare to love that person completely. This dread of parting always hangs in between, a fear that someday they will be going away.

So, instead, we sit there stuck in the middle, holding onto the person for dear life. We sit holding back everything we really want to say. Somehow we cannot dare to be there unreservedly.

But when we can be there completely, parting becomes so much simpler, more natural, and more complete. It is when we have held everything back, waiting for some other moment, that we cannot bear to let him or her go away.

> *When we parted*
> *I thought the autumn*
> *Would dissolve me entirely,*
> *Even the old crows*
> *Outside my window,*
> *Flew away haphazardly.*
>
> Eshin

Underneath all of this fear is grief. What is grief? Where does it come from? How can we recognize it and the odd forms it takes?

For many of us, much of our lives are spent in mourning, weighted down by unconscious grief. We may even be grieving for a person long before he or she has started to leave. Our whole time together, our entire relationship may be a defense against inevitable grief.

A defense is built because we have never learned how to separate, how to be grateful to receive, and then to be willing to say good-bye. In the Jewish religion, when someone dies prayers are repeated for one year. Basically, these are prayers of thankfulness, saying that life is good under all conditions, both when we receive and when we say good-bye.

Moment after moment, we must learn to say good-bye, to allow one thing to be over and then to allow the next to arise anew. Grief is an attempt to hold everything static and in one place. Grief refuses to let go.

Grief can be a deadly weapon. It can work on us in subtle ways beneath the surface, dimming our pleasures, forbidding our success. Grief can be so deep and tenacious that it may even cause illness and death. We may want to stop living; we may feel life is useless. We may be feeling very great rage at having been abandoned, which can turn into grief.

Many mourners die of grief, of a longing to be reunited with a loved one. (There is a high percentage of widows and widowers who die or fall ill after their mate's death). This desire arises out of the sense that I am here, and my loved one is somewhere else, apart from me. I feel I can join him or her by dying myself. This is a very commonplace delusion. It can be quite vivid and compelling.

Some people see their loved ones in familiar places, others hear their voices. Some hold onto their belongings for a very long time. This is not necessarily to be discouraged. It is simply the work of saying good-bye. It is simply the footprints of a griever. We must be allowed to hold onto the person, in whatever way, as long as we need to. When we are ready, we will let them go. Or, allow someone else to come and fill up the void. (We may feel disloyal if we let go too quickly). Or, one day we may begin to realize that the person has not left at all, that he or she is still very much with us in all kinds of wonderful ways.

Process

Think about a loved one you have lost. Do you presently feel him or her with you? In what way?

Grief works in insidious ways, sometimes making us hate ourselves. Some mourners begin to feel that their loved ones left because they were bad, or did not do enough to please him or her. The mourners may feel they never deserved having their loved one there in the first place.

Others may feel as though their thoughts of anger have killed the person. (Children often feel this way; it is crucial to discuss this with them openly, to help make these distinctions for them. They must see that their feelings do not kill another).

These deep, irrational, unconscious responses can truly dominate our lives after the death of a loved one. Some mourners do not eat or wash. Others may seem entirely disoriented. They are. It is alright. Do not press them to be otherwise. They are simply searching for their loved one.

Some may hurt themselves in various ways. There may be a desire for illness or punishment so they, too, can suffer like their loved one. This is a way of staying close to the loved one. Or, of punishing them for going away. ("See how you've hurt me!")

Often there is tremendous guilt for just being alive while the loved one has suffered and died. We may keep ourselves only half-alive, as a kind of penance, or as a kind of identification with loved ones. We are afraid to be too well or happy while our loved ones are dead. In our minds, loved ones may still be suffering, still be in terrible pain. This is all a way to keep loved ones alive. It is a way to join them, pacify them, hold them close to ourselves. These needs and wishes must be respected.

It takes time to realize that the person is not physically here any longer, that we cannot join him or her through our suffering, and that no matter what we do, nothing out there is going to change. Slowly we may realize that our real bond with the person cannot ever go away. It is not our bodies which have become close and united. In death, it is only the body which goes away.

Process

Think of the people you feel truly close to. Where are they now? What makes you feel so connected? If they go away, do you feel less close? When you are together, does that change the essential bond anyway?

Now, think of someone you do not feel so good with. If they are around a lot, do you feel closer? When they go away is your relationship changed?

There are other ways of grieving that are harder to detect and to handle. On the surface, these reactions may not look like grief at all. But they are equally harmful for our well-being and may have unhappy consequences.

It may look as if the mourner is fine now; he or she is going out all the time, running here and there. This may simply be a frantic need to replace the lost person, as if survival itself depended upon the presence of another.

Relationships may be quickly formed, compulsively, to fill the gap. The mourner may be terrified of being alone and experiencing the emptiness. But these new relationships often lack discrimination and care. They are formed by a quality of desperation, and if that new person should go away, all the incomplete mourning for the original loved one will surface suddenly, often in unexpected ways.

The space between two times in life, the *bardo** or passage, is almost unbearable for some. During this period when we are neither here nor there, there is a sense of nondefinition and uncertainty about what will happen. Often there is a sense of loss of moorings, confusion, and fear. This period of transition may seem like it must be avoided. For some it feels like death.

We fear being dead so deeply, we fight it so constantly, that often we do not allow ourselves to experience it at all. Instead we do it indirectly, by sleeping too much, withdrawing, hiding.

Some mourners who withdraw and will not go out anywhere during their mourning are simply in this passage, experiencing death. We must not press them back to life prematurely, but help them go through this journey of death. Going into the darkness, sorrow, and immovability and then returning when we are ready, brings us back refreshed and renewed. We have gone and returned. It takes great courage to allow this journey. If we can go into it deeply, we come back larger and washed clean.

This time of passage, this bardo, is a gift and an offering. It

---

*Francesca Fremantle and Chogyam Trungpa, translators, *Tibetan Book of the Dead* (Berkeley, Calif.: Shambhala, 1975), pp. 1–4.

contains many possibilities. We must trust that someone who undertakes this journey will come back when he or she is ready, when the natural impulse of his or her life draws the person back to it itself.

Here in the West, we have little patience, little understanding of time, process, and transition. Everything here must be accomplished instantly. Like frozen food, the quicker the better. Eat one package, then on to the next thing. We are all in a frenzy.

Mourning and the bardo are times of gestation. They cannot be rushed and pushed through. During true mourning we are being given the opportunity to die also, to let the outworn parts of ourselves vanish. Once they are gone we can grow new and beautiful.

There are many bardo stages that appear during our lifetimes, many opportunities for transition and change. The time of mourning for a loved one is the most intense bardo of all. But we push it away by filling up each moment, and thus withhold this experience from ourselves.

But even though we may refuse to go through this experience, it will return to us over and over until it is complete. Anything that is not completed will return whether we like it or not. The same situation, the same difficulty appears over and over until it has been thoroughly understood.

We are not sure, however, that we want to understand a situation. We are not sure we want to return new and beautiful. Mostly we just want to hold our act together. But at the time of grief and mourning, the more we try to hold our act together, the faster it falls apart.

We are terrified of really mourning. We are taught to be "strong and dignified." There is the idea that it is weak and childish to mourn. Grief can seem uncontrollable, as if it will never have an end.

Nobody wants to be near
A true mourner.
No one will watch
Inappropriate grief.
It is not decent
To walk barefooted
In the winter
Home from the grave,
Stubbing your toes on
The casual pebbles . . .

Eshin

We desperately try to control our feelings. This very effort itself causes the illness and constriction we feel. This causes us to run madly around searching for someone to love. It is healthy, courageous, and strong to grieve. Until we grieve fully, we may not be able to really return back to life again.

If we wish to help someone who is grieving, we must simply help them to honor their feelings. It is foolish to try to cheer them up with superficial gaiety. All of this superficial gaiety can't really be swallowed, sooner or later it comes back up.

It is exhausting, depleting, and finally humiliating to have to constantly put on a front, to have to keep smiling when you are dying inside.

"... I don't want to wear make-up now. I want to cover my face with ashes."
"Alright."
"I don't know who to go to. My therapist is frightened of me. He scrapes his throat, crosses his legs, and wants to analyze my feelings. I only want to scratch out my eyes."
"Alright."

Grief is grief. There is nothing to analyze. It must be experienced and not analyzed. To analyze is to defend against feelings. This gets us nowhere at all with grief.

"Bang the wall, honey! Bang the wall."
"No."
"Bang the wall harder!"
"I hate you."
"Tell the wall everything you hate it for."
"I hate you. I hate you."
"Tell the wall everything you regret."

"Can you love me enough to let me be this ugly?"
"The uglier you are, the more I love you. Just go be as ugly as you want!"

We experience our pain as ugliness. It is not. It can be beautiful too.

I have always looked upon decay as being just as wonderful and rich an expression of life as growth.[2]

Henry Miller

Mourning can end when we are complete; when we have said, done, felt, and expressed whatever is there inside. This may seem like an impossible task. It is not. As soon as we even begin to do this, a wonderful process is set up inside. Then, as soon as we are really complete about even one thing, about even one moment, we feel so full and wonderful that a great deal of our mourning ends right then and there. We feel whole again.

The basic force that keeps mourning going is regret and unfinished business. We have a sense that things are irrevocable, that now we cannot go back and change whatever happened. It's too late! We have done the damage and it cannot be repaired. This is incorrect. Everything can be repaired.

In fact, it is necessary that everything be repaired, in one way or another. We may not be able to change something with a specific person who is gone, but we can learn from the interaction and then make the change (or repair) the next time the situation comes around—and it will. We are always being given opportunities to set things right.

Process

Look at the person you are mourning for. What do you regret most about your relationship? (Make a list of all your regrets.) How do you feel this could be righted? What could you do *now* to make amends? What amends did you make to the person while they were here? (Give yourself credit for it.)

In order to really be able to say good-bye, we have to feel totally complete with another. This means we have to feel as if we have said, done, and experienced with the other all that was there for us to do.

We have let the other person know us truly, and we have truly known the other. The relationship has been fulfilled. We have been the person we wanted to be.

Although we miss the person, we will not mourn him or her so deeply. The person has become part of us now; something vital has been integrated. At first it may seem too frightening, too overwhelming to *complete* a relationship with someone who is dying. You do not know where to begin. You worry about what his or her reaction may be. There may be some sense of futility, as if no matter what you say or do, it won't really change anything anyway. He or she won't hear you. It's just too late.

It is never too late to complete a relationship. At every moment we have the opportunity to be the person we always wanted to be. Just one moment of being real and truthful begins to dissolve the pain of the past. And, it does not matter if another does or does not hear you. Your own act of truthfulness releases you from a sense of pain no matter what his or her reaction may be.

If the other person hears and responds, certainly that is wonderful. Even if he or she cannot, it is still wonderful. You have done what had to be done. You will feel different irregardless, and in some subtle way, he or she will too.

When you are able to do this with a loved one before he or she dies, your process of mourning will be very much different.

Start simply by telling the other person what he or she has meant to you and what he or she gave you in your life. Tell the other person what you wanted from him or her; find the good things, discuss the problems.

It never helps anyone to keep negative feelings and thoughts tucked down deep inside. When they are brought to the surface, shared, and understood, then we can be finished with them and have much more room for the love which is there to emerge. Usually we are afraid to express anger and disappointment. Anger and disappointment are only another part of love. You cannot have one without the other.

> . . . *Eve had been dying for three months now and I was exhausted and furious. Every morning I woke up furious, I dreaded the day, I dreaded seeing her. All of my anger just stared me in the face. It was always there like a huge block between us. I'd been angry with Eve for a very long*

time anyway, and there she was now, in front of me dying. I felt like she was getting me back.

I was terrified of my feelings. I was terrified of what I might be doing to her. But it was there anyway, like a boulder between us. It stopped anything nice from happening. Every day we just looked at each other blankly.

So, finally, one day I sat down near her and I just cried. It was all too much. I cried and I cried. I knew she was frightened, but I told her, 'I'm sorry Eve, but I'm so angry with you. And I'm frightened too. Oh God, I'm so frightened.'

Then, thank God, she started crying too. It felt so good, the both of us crying. It was really a great relief to me. Before she just lay there like a clay statue. At least she was crying now, at least she was alive.

Then I took her in my arms and hugged her. For the first time I could really hug her and feel how much she meant to me.

Mrs. Aubin, mother of a dying child

The very act of telling someone that we are angry or frightened by them, that very act is an act of love and true appreciation. The other person knows it anyway. It is impossible not to be moved when someone is being truthful with us. It is impossible not to feel loved.

On the other hand, our falseness and lies are often experienced as a kind of withdrawal. This withdrawal itself contributes so much to the pain and loneliness we feel. We think we are protecting each other by playing some kind of a role, but the kind of numbness it creates is the worst kind of pain of all.

The worst thing of all is to lay there blocked out. They come in and stare. They see you as if you were already dead, and then they say platitudes that mean nothing to you. They mean nothing to them either. You want to shout out. I'm not dead, son-of-a-bitch. I have feelings; I have a heart. I want someone to hold me close and tell me everything they really feel. Oh God, I pray, just let them be real.

Peter, a twenty-seven-year-old man dying of heart disease

In order to understand a little more deeply what it means to complete a relationship, we will do a process to explore it. This kind of process is very valuable, not only with people who are dying, but with everyone in our lives. If we can learn to relate this way on an on-going basis, our entire lives can open up.

Process

Have a friend read the following instructions softly to you.

Close your eyes, relax, become comfortable. You are now in a very beautiful place. Picture it. It is a place that you feel safe, at home, and comfortable in. Picture yourself there, walking in the setting.

Now, picture someone you love who is dying (or dead). Bring him or her to you. Have him or her sit beside you. What do you want to say to him or her? Think back over your time together. What has been left unsaid? Can you say it now?

Let him or her answer you now. What does the person want to reply to you? What is the most beautiful thing you remember between both of you? Tell him or her. What is it that you would like to change? What are you still wanting from him or her? What have you left to give, or to do?

Take a moment now, and realize that the person is about to go away. What needs to happen between both of you in order for you to feel peaceful and complete with him or her? What has to happen for you to be able to let him or her go? Can you let it happen? If not, can you talk about it with him or her? Is there something you want the person to do or say to you, in order for you to be able to let him or her go? Can you ask the person for it?

Now, picture the person leaving. Picture yourself letting him or her go. How do you feel now? What has he or she left you with? What has the person taken away? Perhaps you would like to make a drawing of it.

As you do this process, old feelings of sadness or failure, anger or pain, may emerge. Do not be afraid of them. Let them emerge and then let them go.

Underneath all of the pain, there is always love and forgiveness waiting. It may not seem that way momentarily, but inevitably it is so. You cannot get to that, however, until you experience what is in the way. It may not always be pleasant.

As soon as we have forgiven a person and received his or her forgiveness in return, then all is settled. Mourning is over. Only the love between us remains.

We cannot avoid asking for forgiveness and giving it in return.

If we do not do this, we may spend years after his or her death occupied in self-punishment.

Process

Ask for forgiveness for whatever it is that you did (or think you did) to hurt the person. Offer him or her your forgiveness in return for whatever he or she did that might have hurt you.

The very act of forgiveness is so healing that it may restore some back to health immediately. At the very least, it will greatly ease a variety of discomforts.

At first you may feel that forgiveness is just impossible between you and the other person, but this is when we grieve the most. There is a tremendous amount of rage locked into mourning, rage against the other person and against yourself. By not forgiving, we are simply holding onto the rage, holding onto the person in a negative way.

Process

In a case like this, when we are both locked into anger, it is helpful to begin to list all of the lovely things the person ever did for you. Or that he or she ever did for someone else. Make a conscious effort to find the goodness in the person. It is there, and if you cannot find it, then the block exists in you and not in the other person.

Now, also find your own beauty and goodness. Make a list of all the wonderful things you did for that person (or for another). Tell the other person about it. Tell the person how happy and proud you are of him or her and of yourself. Congratulate each other.

It is often so much easier to find fault, to hate ourselves and others, to feel ashamed and inadequate. These kinds of feelings are commonplace and familiar. We seem to love to dwell on them. It is much easier to forget or gloss over the wonderful things about us and others.

This can be consciously reversed. Dwell upon the ways in which you helped, loved, and cheered the other person. What wonderful things can you do for him or her now? Are you willing to? Why not? What do you think that he or she really needs from you? Does it feel better to stay locked in revenge? Revenge backfires. You are more hurt by it than the other person.

When we love someone, we do not have to possess him or her, the love is there forever. When we are open and truthful with someone, then we can let him or her go. Although the other person may go, his or her love stays with us. Some have even had the sense that the relationship lasts throughout eternity.

> *I always loved you, even before I knew you. Now that I have met you, I know that I met you only so I could see how much I loved you. This love was always there for you.*
>
> *Just even knowing you for a little, we have said everything already. My death cannot take anything away. You did not come to me, and you cannot leave me. We are together for eternity.*

Andrea, from a letter to her boyfriend

> *Three times it cried*
> *And was heard no more,*
> *The voice of the deer.*

Zen poem

part two
BUILDING BRIDGES

On the road, the traveller walks endlessly...

Eshin

Our entire life consists of building bridges. Bridges from where? To where? Who is the traveller and where is he or she going? In the misty night, it is often not so easy to see. On the clear morning, the sun shines blindingly. It may be easier to stay lost in the forest.

Our life is also a bridge. Each person we meet may be another bridge, another link, a new way to deepen the love and under-standing we become capable of. Being together, the bridge grows and develops. The bridge between two people is the most important bridge of all. Yet, so few of us know how to build this, so few allow it, or if we do, it is only for a few precious moments, and then we quickly run away and hide.

In a sense, we are all like flowers longing for the light and sun while we keep our petals shut. There is plenty of sun and plenty of light, but we are keeping ourselves closed tightly. Nobody else can open you up.

The crucial kind of bridge is the one which draws one person, one being toward another. This bridge must cross many kinds of obstacles. Our first response to the other person is usually suspicion, rejection, or some kind of criticism. There is an automatic response against becoming close.

What really is needed to build a bridge of true communication? What happens to tear it down? Why do we often come away from one another hurting, lonely, and filled with misunderstandings?

Without a bridge from person to person, life becomes empty and meaningless. All the things you buy in the world cannot fill it up.

Communication is a massive topic. And yet, nothing really can be said in words. Out of the silence comes the deepest communication. But to begin with, we start out with words.

Basically, there is nothing but communication streaming around us endlessly. And yet most of us live in solitude, hearing noise and not communication. This noise can become so intense and brutal that we find more and more ways of shutting it out. Most of us live large portions of our lives in blindness and deafness, shutting the world out. This shut-upness can become so severe that neurosis and psychosis, as well as distortions of all kinds, commonly develop.

In order to set things right once again, we need only allow the world back in. When we allow ourselves to receive the world, to receive its true communication, much illness and confusion will fade away.

Why do we not allow this to happen? We are so afraid to see, hear, and realize what is going on around us. We fear it may be too much for us to handle and we may be overwhelmed. We do so many things to stave off the contact. We meet another person and label him or her immediately. Instead of being a person, he or she is just another thing; a patient, stranger, or opponent. Judging and labelling this way, we are constantly separating ourselves from the other person. Placing ourselves thus in our own little prisons, we begin to wonder why we feel so alone.

Loneliness, separation, and a deep sense of estrangement make up the real illness of our times. This itself is a cancer, a cancer that becomes clearly manifest during the time of illness and death. At this time when the need for contact is most vital, we instead find withdrawal and lies. The withdrawal is so pervasive that it is even taken for the norm, even encouraged. Drugs are offered routinely. We beg for anesthesia and oblivion.

Instead of being fully present, we put ourselves and our loved ones to sleep. We are pushing life away, with all of its experiences, the pain as well as the joy. By withdrawing from the pain, we are also withdrawing from the love and the beauty.

It may take a while to see that by abandoning our experience, we are also abandoning those we love.

It has been said that if you can touch and be touched truly, then all sickness and pain goes away.

What does this mean?

chapter five
Communication

... *Who is willing to risk being truthful with me? Let him come up here, and I'll give him all my money.*

... *Don't worry, madam. Your husband is in a coma.*

... *Oh, if he's in a coma, then I'll be truthful. He can't hear me anyway!*

Just as the most eager speaking at one another does not make a conversation, so for a true conversation, no sound is necessary, not even a gesture.[1]

Buber

What is communication? There is so much spoken and written on this topic that we may feel saturated even before we begin. Yet, this is the essence of our existence, the need to be known, seen, and understood; the need to be in true touch with others.

Many complain that they are not understood. Wives feel that their husbands do not *communicate*. Nurses feel that doctors do not *communicate*. Patients feel that the medical staff does not *communicate*. Families have their own intricate ways of communicating, and often dedicate all their efforts to keeping each other from knowing the truth.

[1]Excerpts from Martin Buber, *Between Man and Man*, Copyright © 1965 by Macmillan Publishing Co., Inc. Used by permission of Macmillan Publishing Co., Inc., and Routledge & Kegan Paul, Ltd.

There are as many different ways of communicating as there are people, and there are just as many different ways of listening and being heard.

For some, their lives are dedicated to not communicating through hiding, withholding, and presenting a front. These individuals live in a prison of their own making.

There are no gifted and ungifted here, only those who give themselves and those who withhold.[2]

Buber

All fronts are really transparent anyway. We all see through one another, although we are unwilling to admit this easily. But no matter how much we play-act with one another, our deeper communications are always being heard, and always being responded to. It cannot be any other way. Not being willing to communicate is a kind of communication too.

Process

When do you communicate most fully? Who are you most willing to communicate with? Who are you unwilling to communicate with? Why? What's the difference? How do *you* feel in both instances?

Throughout most of our lives, we all play a variation of the game, "Let's Pretend." Let's pretend that you are King Arthur and I am the Queen. Let's pretend that you didn't say that and that I didn't hear you. I help you keep your pretenses up and you help me keep up mine. Now we all feel safe and secure.

The only thing is, we are living in a make-believe world. We become cardboard people, papier-mache, unreal. If we knock on the door it can fall down because there is really nobody home. When someone is dying and they knock on our door, they need a real person to hold onto. There is no more pretending when we come to death. This is for real. We want a real hand to hold.

The best preparation for work with the dying is to work with

[2]Buber, *Between Man and Man.*

yourself, to become a real person. This may not be so easy at first. Everyone fears being exposed. This seems to be one of the greatest fears of all. Some would rather die on the spot than have their masks taken off. Many dying are still primarily concerned with how they look to others, about the impression they will make. But death itself wipes out all images, removes all masks and games.

Who am I when I have no body remaining? What is it that we are so afraid of exposing, of knowing, of seeing about ourselves? What is it that we are so afraid of responding to?

Being completely involved in presenting a front to others, we lose touch with who we truly are. When our entire attention is riveted to the outside, we become trapped in another's eyes. This prevents true communication. We are still completely tied up with our own small self.

Communication has many facets. We talk and listen in many ways. At the uppermost layer, there is what we are saying in words. Then, beneath that, there is our body language, the messages our movements make. How do we stand, sit, move, gesture? How are we dressed? These two types of communication can easily get mixed up.

Process

Say, "I love you," without using words. Say, "Go away," without using words. Say one thing with words and the opposite with your body language.

Play with these actions for a while. It is very important to become aware of the discrepant communication that we continually make. Are we using our communication to be in touch with the other, or are we using it to hide? Or, to confuse and mystify?

Why are we communicating after all? What is our purpose and intention? There are many different kinds of communication that we make.

We may communicate in order to express our feelings, to unburden ourselves. "I love you, I hate you, I hate you, I love you." (Think of examples of some of these kinds of communication.) Or, we may simply wish to deliver a message. There may be something specific to convey. "Dinner will be ready at five."

We may be communicating in order to influence the other, to

control, or elicit a certain kind of response. "You look so beautiful tonight." What is behind this communication? Do we want warmth back? Do we want to hold the affection of the other? It can also be quite clear that we want something explicit from the other. "I want you to tell me the truth—and now!"

Or, suddenly, we may allow our heart to speak out all by itself. Our hearts have a language of their own. The voice of the heart is always eager to speak out from within, while we always try to suppress it. Sometimes it bursts out all by itself. In the highest form, this turns into prayer.

Process

Find a partner and try out each of the above types of communication with him or her. (The four types of communication are: to express our feelings, to deliver a message, to influence another, to allow our hearts to speak by themselves.) How do you feel in each instance? How does he or she feel? How is he or she responding to you?

Contained in the way in which we speak to another is our entire relation to him or her. It may not be our words the person is responding to, but our relation to him or her. Implicitly, no matter what we say, we are communicating what the other person means to us, who he or she is in our world.

The other person may mean nothing to us; we may speak to him or her as if he or she were an object, a table or chair, existing for our purposes with no feelings of its own at all. This is a highly impersonal communication, delivered in a highly impersonal manner. (Some may say "I love you" in just this way.)

In a situation such as this, the person spoken to will shrivel up inside, feeling bossed, lectured, or pushed around. In severe cases, he or she may even directly experience him- or herself as an object and not feel alive or well at all. This kind of communication drains away life and enthusiasm. It does not produce wellness or joy. The person feels as if he or she does not matter, and the person is right. In your world, he or she really does not. He or she is only an object to you. Unfortunately, some patients have this experience with doctors; so do some nurses. A person's own family or family members may treat him or her in this manner as well. It is extremely important to be aware of this behavior and of the response it creates.

Process

Talk to another as if he or she were a chair, an object to be moved around, which is only there to serve you. Now, let yourself be talked to that way. How does it feel? What kind of inner response are you having, no matter what the person is saying in *words*? Say "I love you" to a person in this manner. Let him or her say it to you. How does it feel? What do you want to really reply to the other person?

There is another way in which we can relate to another person. In this way, we are fully aware that the other is also a person, that he or she is alive and has feelings of his or her own. Our experience of the person makes room for his or her responses. We can allow the other person to be there as he or she really is; not as we demand he or she be in order to suit our own purposes. In this kind of relationship we are able to tolerate the other person being different from us. We can allow the other person to respond to us in his or her own time and way. This kind of relationship can develop into dialogue.

In the first kind of relationship, no real communication is possible. The only thing possible is that we use the other person to fulfill our own desires.

In the second kind of relationship, we are opening ourselves up to something different, to something *other* than we are. This can feel dangerous because it is unpredictable. We may feel as if something uncontrollable is about to take place. In this kind of relationship, we do not so much need to control. Here there is a possibility of a real meeting.

What is a real meeting? What is true communication? How do we know when it is happening?

A real meeting takes us home to our center. There is no more wandering, lost and alone. Our sense of alienation vanishes. We see that we are truly one.

This real meeting can happen suddenly, spontaneously. It can happen for a moment, or it can last. It can happen between two people, or between a person and the sky, the birds, anything. We cannot demand that a real meeting happen, but we can invite it. There are various ways.

First, we must see what prevents it, and then what is required for a real meeting to take place. The most important ingredients are two real people. This requires that each person be willing, in that moment, to let go of his or her need to control the other, to use the other person for his or her own selfish desires. It requires that we completely forget about using the other person as a table or chair.

We must also forget about our own self-affirmation. In that moment, we must also forget about wanting praise in the other person's eyes. We do not have to be important, wonderful, or special in any way. We simply have to *be*. That is the most wonderful of all. Here we are not using the relation as a way to develop our own fantasy about who we are. We are really not *using* the relation for anything. We are simply willing to be present for each moment and able to allow anything to happen, exactly as it wants to be. For that time, we forget about fear and about protecting ourselves. We may even see that there is nothing to protect, except our own fantasy. This kind of meeting is tremendously liberating. Many begin to laugh out loud, or to cry, but they are tears of wonder.

Most of us have experienced a taste of this kind of meeting at one time or another. It is everyone's natural birthright.

In order to fully court this kind of meeting, this kind of interaction, we need to prepare ourselves and continually make ourselves ready. It is as if we were constantly preparing ourselves to go in to visit a great king.

Martin Buber describes this kind of meeting beautifully in his essay, "Between Man and Man." Here two strangers meet in the early evening on a deserted platform, waiting for a train. They know nothing of one another, but sit beside one another. One is reading his newspaper. The train arrives and the two enter the train, sit together, and do not speak. Suddenly, unexpectedly, full communication streams from one person to the other. During this time each knows everything about the other. They feel as close to one another as to their very selves. Both hearts have opened and spoken to one another, although not a word has been said.

What is this? Buber says it is as though a spell were lifted and the reserve which we usually hold over ourselves is released, which allows a true meeting to take place.

It is this kind of interaction and this kind of preparation which is needed in working with the dying. Many of the dying are more ready for this. They are more open than we are, more available. Being closer to death, they have less to hold on to. Their time is shorter. Their need greater. This is a very special opportunity. It is not enough to go into their rooms and talk about the weather.

To start our preparation for this kind of meeting, we must first look at that which gets in our way. How do our opinions, needs and intentions intrude upon our communication with the other?

Process

Two partners are required for this exercise. One person is A, the other is B.

First we will look at how it feels to make the various kinds of communication we are used to. We will begin to become conscious of what we are doing. Until we become conscious about what is going on, there is no possibility of change. In all communication, A will communicate and B will receive the communication. B, notice how you are feeling when you are being communicated to in various ways. What kind of response do you want to make? (During the actual exercise, do not respond, but discuss your responses after it is over.)

A, communicate something to B as if he or she was completely unimportant to you.

A, communicate something to B with the intention of making him or her like you.

A, communicate something to B that he or she will have difficulty hearing, something that would seem strange and disturbing to him or her.

A, communicate something intimate to B, something that is true and important to you.

A, just be there with B. Experience whatever it is you are feeling inside. Find some way to share it with him or her.

Now, reverse roles and repeat the exercise.

B's role is extremely important too. What does it mean to really listen? What gets in the way? How much of the time was B able to really listen?

It is difficult to communicate when you do not feel anyone is there listening to you. Sometimes when we are listening we do not hear the other person, but only our own response to what was said. Sometimes the other person simply stirs up our own fantasies, and our fantasies get between us and him or her.

When you are listening, notice your responses to the following questions.

Did you have feelings about what was being said? Did these feelings get in the way?

Were you busy making judgments of the other person? Did these judgments get in the way?

Did you feel a compulsion to express your feelings and opinions? To set this person straight? This isn't listening. It's bulldozing.

Did you want to impress the other person with how silent and thoughtful you were? This isn't listening either. It's just trying to create an impression.

Look at the person speaking closely. Who is this other person to you?

Can you completely release this individual from your need to have him or her be any particular way?

Can you love this person just as he or she is?

It is rare and wonderful to have an experience of someone listening to you deeply, of being really heard. When we have this experience, we truly feel loved.

As we prepare for the real meeting, we move onto another kind of communication. This is a completely nonverbal communication. It is the communication we receive just being in the presence of another. Nothing extra has to be said or done.

Around some people we feel joyous and loved, there may be no particular reason why. We find we just want to be around these individuals, that there is a sense of well-being here. Around others, we feel tight and constricted. Perhaps we want to run away. Again, there may be no particular reason that we can point to.

Around some people plants grow wildly. Around others, they wither and die. Why? What is the reason? Plants don't need a reason, they do not ask any questions. They just bloom or die. Plants are simply responding. Like the plants, despite all our reasons, we just bloom or wither too. We are also always responding. Often we are trained to overlook this fundamental internal response we are having.

All our lives we have been trained to mistrust this inner responding. Instead, we are taught to find evidence for what we feel and what we do. We are taught to turn to the objective world to come to our conclusions. We are supposed to like someone because of his or her merits and dislike someone because of his or her faults. But it doesn't work this way. Deep down we love the villains and don't really feel good near the so-called saints. Another kind of communication is happening. No matter what we are thinking, we are always in touch with each other in a different kind of way too.

It is this different kind of communication that we must develop around the dying. This is the kind of communication that makes plants grow and makes us feel full inside. It is this kind of communication that the dying are in touch with as the outside world is slipping away.

We go to great lengths to deny this kind of communication. For some it seems very confusing because we have been taught to confuse communication with *consensual validation*.

Consensual validation is based upon the outside world. Consensual validation says, "my perceptions and feelings are true only if everyone else agrees with them too. If not, I must be strange, crazy, or undependable. I need the group to check myself out. I'd better analyze myself to find out what I am feeling."

This kind of attitude is valid in science. It is part of the objective inquiry process. But at the bedside of someone who is dying, it is absolutely irrelevant. At the bedside of the dying, we must have the utmost respect and care for our own unique experience, and also for theirs.

Generally, we have not learned how to honor our experience, to welcome our uniqueness. We have been taught to feel ashamed and analyze what we are feeling, to make ourselves like everyone else. This is a form of suicide, self-rejection, a way to apologize for who we are.

Rather than be true to our own feelings, we feel we must be accepted by everyone else, to live all together on one plateau. But when someone is very ill or dying, he or she is travelling from one plateau to another. What difference can it possibly make to him or her then what everybody else is feeling? The person simply needs you to honor him or her and his or her experience, and to honor your own. Are you willing to take this journey with him or her?

At the bedside of the dying, a change in emphasis is required. We must be willing to honor, accept, and recognize our own experience, as well as that of the dying person. Dying people may feel quite lonely and alienated because they are having an experience that they feel is different and that they cannot share with others. They may be seeing, hearing, or knowing things that they may feel afraid to share.

A person who is dying often becomes more and more sensitive, more intuitive. He or she may begin to feel and to see more than ever before. Old feelings and memories often surface. That which has been incomplete may return again, so he or she can come to terms with it. Although this feels strange, it can also be very beautiful. A kind of flow now begins to happen. Sometimes these memories are experienced visually. From the outside we label them hallucinations. But that is only a label. The label implies that they are not true. They *are* true for the dying person, and not only are they true, it is also quite possible that the dying may be seeing *more* clearly and fully than we are at that moment. Many of the dying often know more than we do about their own condition, such as exactly when they will die. (They may receive this information up to several weeks before they die). It is presumptuous to try to analyze exactly what is happening, or to try to dismiss anyone's experience.

The best way is to stay away from all labels and need to grasp the situation *intellectually*. Instead, simply *be there* and be open, accepting, and fully available to whatever is going on. This kind of attitude and state of being will bring the deepest sense of comfort and well-being to all concerned.

Medical personnel and families often ask the same question: "Should we tell the truth to the dying?" This question itself is basically ridiculous. The dying know that they are dying. You are not asking about the dying, you are asking about yourself. The real question is not, "Should I tell the truth to the dying?" The real question is, "Am I willing to openly face and deal with what is going on?" That is a legitimate question. You have every right to ask it and every right to answer it in any way that you feel able.

Look at *yourself* carefully and see, can *you* handle it? Are you willing to enter into an honest, open exchange with this person, or would you rather keep your distance? This is a choice you have to make.

If the person who is dying is asking you for information and you feel reluctant to give it, please consider the following for a moment. This person is asking for clarity. Do you have the right to withhold that? Does this information "belong" to you? Whose life is it? Do you have the right to decide for another what he or she should or should not experience? These are questions that each one of us must answer. There is no ready-made answer in any textbook. Each person must come to terms with it for him- or herself. The most we can do is offer the questions, clearly and directly, for *you* to answer.

Process

While you are struggling with these questions, just think for a moment: Do you want to know the truth about *your* condition? Are you protecting the other person because you would want to be protected someday? What is the value both of you could derive from dealing with the truth together? What are the difficulties?

Write down the answers to these questions. Do not gloss over them in a hurried way. Spend some time really considering them. You might even wish to pretend that you are dying and write a spontaneous letter to a friend telling him or her what you want during this time of your life.

Whichever choice you make, whether or not to deal openly with the dying, just be clear and honest about it. Either choice is acceptable, as long as it is dealt with directly. What is not so acceptable is when we engage in mystification.

Mystification is another form of communication. Unfortunately, this is common around the dying. This term describes the efforts (conscious or unconscious) of one person to confuse, mystify, or deny the feelings and perceptions of another. It is a kind of communication that obscures and clouds the truth. The person who is being mystified has the sense of not having any solid ground to stand on. He or she may be receiving two opposing types of communication simultaneously. We say one thing with words and the opposite nonverbally. The person does not know which communication to respond to. This kind of communication causes paralysis. It is the best way to drive someone crazy, including yourself, and to feel out of touch with reality.

SUSAN: Whenever I want to come close and touch you, you pull away.
MOTHER: I do not.
SUSAN: Yes, you do. I feel it.
MOTHER: Look. I am standing right here.
SUSAN: You are not here. You are far away. You are a thousand miles away from me.
MOTHER: (crying) I am not a thousand miles away. I am right here. I am right here. See. See.
SUSAN: I am looking, but I can't see.

Susan, a nine-year-old girl dying, to her mother

What is happening in this beautiful, poignant dialogue? Susan is crying out for her mother to come close to her inside. Her mother is keeping her distance. She must be afraid, as she is standing very far away. (There are two levels of reality taking place here. On the external level, her mother is there. On the internal level, she is far away.)

Some reading this interchange would immediately wish to deny, explain, and analyze Susan's perception. That misses the point entirely. First of all, there is no denying Susan's perception. If her mother were close (inside), Susan would feel it. Susan's feelings (perceptions) must be accepted, although they may differ from what we see outside. Susan is responding on the level of plants. She is just feeling. She wants the sun. Her mother does not offer the warmth. Her mother is standing in the shade.

On the level of external, objective reality, her mother is there. Her body is there. But where is her mother really? The mother keeps pointing only to this level of reality, the external level, saying, "Look, I am here." However, this level is *not* sufficient now. Also, it is very confusing for Susan. It does *seem* as if her mother were there, but still she feels that her mother is very far away. When one is very ill or dying, one becomes tuned to the internal levels. The outside world is slipping away. Our inner experience is stronger and sharper and it predominates.

Some psychologists would say that this child is experiencing feelings of separation and loneliness and is then *projecting* these feelings onto the mother. The crucial word here is *projecting*, as this word implies that the child is simply placing her own inner world out onto another. It does not include the fact that the child is responding to the inner world of the other person too.

Actually, in truth, both activities are going on simultaneously. But, for now, our necessary focus must be upon the other person, upon the ways in which the mother can be with the child so that feelings of loneliness and estrangement subside.

The mother must start by acknowledging that probably she *is* running away inside. If she could share this feeling with her child, her child would be relieved tremendously. (That in itself would bring them much closer.)

In this case, the mother becomes involved in defending herself. By defending herself, she is rejecting the child's experience. She is not willing to allow the child to have *her* experience and to validate it.

Just to allow the child's experience, to validate it, would give the child what she needed. However, the mother does not do this. At this moment, the mother *is* pushing the child away.

There are many distances that must be crossed by the dying. At this time, some feel the distance between themselves and another very strongly. However, when the other person is available with acceptance and love, the dying also feel that very strongly.

When our posturing and pretense have subsided, then presense and love can arise. All pretense means nothing to the dying. It is absolutely essential to let it subside. The art of truly communicating is the art of getting out of the way, of not being afraid, of allowing ourselves to be who we truly are and allowing the other person too.

When we retreat into roles and games, the words we say will be empty. Others will listen and not believe them. Our sense of trust and our sense of union will be constantly impaired.

To learn the art of communication is simply to learn how to love.

All I ever wanted from you, Mother, was for you to know me just as I
was and to feel that I was wonderful.
... Even now, this very moment, I still want that from you.
Can you give it to me?

Andrea, a seventeen-year-old girl dying from leukemia

chapter six
Role-Playing

Give up sirs, your proud airs, your many wishes, mannerisms and extravagant claims. They won't do you any good, sir! That's all I have to tell you.

Lao Tse

IMAGES, MIRAGES, DREAMS

In order to deepen our understanding of communication, we must look more closely at the roles we play. These roles, dreams, and images are often what get in the way of truly knowing each other.

I want to communicate who I truly am, but how do I discover who I am, today, tomorrow, an hour from now? When asked, "Who am I?" how do I identify myself?

Process

Who are you? Describe yourself.

Who am I?
   "I'm beautiful, young, and slender. The whole universe belongs to me."
Who do you belong to?
   "I belong to myself."

70

"I belong to my father."
"I belong to my mother."
"I don't belong anywhere."
What are you committed to?
"I'm committed to wealth."
"I'm committed to pleasure."
"I'm committed to working tremendously hard."
"I'm committed to God."
How do you know who you are?
"I'm a doctor. I'm extremely successful, handsome, and strong. I have respect wherever I go."
"I'm a mother. My children love me."
"I'm a dancer. When I dance, then I know."
"I'm a robot. I do what I'm told to do."
"If I look beautiful, then I'm okay."

We wear many hats. In each hat we look and feel slightly different. These hats are comfortable. They keep off the wind, the snow, and the rain. Sometimes a hat you wear gets stuck to your head. You don't remember that you have just put it on for the afternoon. You begin to admire this hat that you wear and forget that your face is hidden beneath it.

During a time of illness and loss, especially in a hospital or any kind of medical establishment, the reality that is going on is so disturbing and so frightening, that we automatically dress up and begin to play our roles. These roles give us a sense of temporary security. Temporary security isn't bad, but it is only temporary and does not deal with the inner turbulence. Sooner or later this turbulence emerges. It is really much better to look closely at the roles we play and the ways in which they do or do not serve us.

Roles can be hypnotic. We can fall in love with a role or fantasy and begin to believe that it is who we truly are. Or, more commonly, we can fall in love with someone who is playing out a role. (Are we falling in love with the person or with the image he or she is creating for us?) It can come as quite a shock when the person puts his or her role away and we are face-to-face with someone quite different.

Patients can easily become mesmerized by the role the physician plays. It is easy to begin to believe that this person is really in total command of the situation, of the patient's life, and even perhaps of the universe. It may be comforting to feel there is someone out there who knows everything, especially while patients are feeling so shaky. Then we put ourselves at their mercy. Many patients gladly give away their own power and independence, easily relinquishing their decision-making ability, in exchange for such powerful care.

Does this work to the best advantage of the patient or the physician? Some would argue that it works to everyone's best advantage. This argument is a viable one that needs to be brought out into the open and discussed thoroughly. We must become aware of both sides of the story.

All roles are based on appearances, images, and dreams. These images tap into our secret longings and address parts of ourselves that may be unconscious. We may be responding not to the reality, but to our own secret dreams and needs. We can become so involved in the roles we are playing, and the effect they are having on others, that we lose touch with what really is going on at that moment, in that particular situation. We may not be able to see the full range of possibilities that exist for us.

Roles limit and define the possibilities of our behaviors. Certain kinds of responses are expected when we play certain kinds of roles. If we become too wedded to the role-image, we may not be able to see what is most suitable in a given moment. The role may begin to play us, rather than vice-versa. At these times we are no longer of maximal help to our patients, friends, or family members.

ROLES

A *role* is a set of behaviors intended to project a certain kind of image to others and to ourselves. In each role we adopt certain behaviors, feelings, and attitudes that are a given part of the role. These responses are built in automatically. Within each role there are also a set of behaviors that we would consider out of order. For instance, we would be startled if our physician started to cry. Our physician would be startled too, and might even feel he or she was falling apart. The physician might not be aware that this particular behavior could be the best thing at the moment for him or her *and* the patient. Usually we do not consider behavior outside of the role as possible for us to engage in. When we do, we call ourselves sick, bad, or confused.

Process

What kind of behaviors do you feel are off-limits for you in the the roles you have adopted? How does this affect your over-all functioning?

The limitation on acceptable behavior causes an inner feeling of entrapment, burn-out, and boredom that many professionals feel. This kind of feeling most often comes upon us when our lives are mostly involved in performing gestures instead of acts.

ACTS AND GESTURES

A *gesture* looks like an act. It is the outward expression of an act, but springs from a different source. A gesture is not spontaneous. It is a proscribed part of the entire role. It is the "right and proper" thing to do. It is expected, regulated, predictable behavior. While a gesture is the outward form, an act is the inner meaning.

An *act* emerges from somewhere else. It is spontaneous, vital, and corresponds to the moment. It does not necessarily correspond to some preconceived image of how we should behave. All acts, which arise out of the depth of our being, are healing. They cannot be otherwise. When we perform an act as opposed to a gesture, we are speaking from deep within, and that is how we are being heard by another. This will make an impression far beyond that which we might have imagined simply by playing a role. When an act happens, it feels full, balanced, and absolutely appropriate to the moment. We feel as if the moment had been responded to completely. This is what we are all capable of.

BEING

We say that true acts arise out of the depth of our Being. What does this mean? Existentialists speak a great deal about Being, about the deep, open flow of existence. This natural, open flow, which is available to everyone, can become hampered and cut off. Why?

Because we do not use it, reach for it, love it, and live out of the flow. We live instead out of the fixed images created by our roles.

The natural, open flow of existence has no fixed roles. Everything moves, everything changes. We are here one moment, and there the next. Most of us are afraid of this movement, so we live our lives predictably, encased within our roles. We feel stifled, lifeless, bored with ourselves and each other, and wonder why. We live more like machines than like true men and women. What does it mean to be a true man or woman?

> *A true man belongs to no time or place, but is the center of things. Where he is, there is nature.*
>
> Ralph Waldo Emerson

For many of us the idea of being *true* has become confused with the idea of being selfish, and not caring about the feelings of the other. Oddly enough, just the opposite is so. When we are able to respond truly, we help the other to do this too. Our way of being strikes a chord deep within our friend. This chord reverberates in many wonderful ways inside. It is ultimately healing to be with someone who is willing to be true. It allows us the same privilege and much of the pain we feel in relationships disappears all by itself.

On the other hand, when we act from our roles, we are implicitly demanding this kind of preconceived response from the other. This kind of relating can be very deadening, as we become so marvellous at manipulating each other. Then we wonder why we feel so relieved when the other goes away.

Process

Look for a moment at what being a "true man or woman" means to you.

The way we act, the nature of our responding, inevitably creates a response in the other. For every role we play there is a complementary part that the other must play in return. Just by virtue of the roles we choose, we create the others' behavior around us.

For every mother, there must be a child.
For every physician, there must be a patient.
For every tyrannical person, there must be someone who wants to be tyrannized.

Process

What roles do you love to play? Take a look at the roles you play regularly. Write them down. Which ones do you enjoy the most? Which roles are you afraid of?

Pick the role you like the best. Now, find a partner and play it out a little with him or her. How do you feel right now, playing it? What kind of response is it creating in your partner? Ask your partner.

Now, reverse roles. Have your partner play out your role. How do you feel on the other side of it? Do you like it? Who are you without a role? Who are you without somebody to play with?

All of this is not implying that we should never play roles. Life demands that we play many roles, and versatility in role-playing is required of all of us. The problem is not with playing a role, the problem is when we become so identified with a role that we lose touch with what is truly fulfilling.

We can play roles for many different reasons. We can play a role in order to hide our feelings. Or, we can play a role in order to dominate another, and then simply blame it on the role. ("This is how mothers *have to* behave. If I didn't punish him, then I wouldn't be a good mother.") Look and see how you are using the different roles that you play.

Some feel completely trapped into a role, or trapped (intimidated) by the strong roles others around them are playing. They do not see that they always have the option of simply redefining the role at any time at all. (Often a marriage will break up because the partners do not realize that they have the option of re-defining their roles, playing it differently).

It always take two players to keep a scene going. You cannot be a mother without someone who wants to be mothered. You cannot be a wonderful physician without someone who is very sick.

ROLE DEFINITION

A role is defined by the complementary player. The weaker I am, the stronger you become. Each person's part is inextricably interwoven with the other person's. The mother and child, the physician and patient, are dancing the same steps together. One is leading and the other is following, but they have both chosen to do the same dance.

If one day you no longer want to do the tango, you may go and find a partner to do the waltz. There are an infinite number of dances to do, an infinite number of roles to choose from. Within each role there are an infinite number of ways to play.

We are *not* the roles we have chosen. At one point we chose them and now we can choose to throw them away. Or, better yet, we can choose to redefine them.

Who has defined these roles in the first place? *Who* is agreeing to play them each day? What stops you right now from finding an entirely new definition to the roles you play? Also look carefully at the benefits you are receiving from playing a particular role.

Process

Make a list of the major roles you are playing. How do you define and describe them? What kinds of behaviors, attitudes, and responses are expected from you?

Now, turn it around. Define the role in an entirely different way. Try it out. Find a partner and play it out with him or her.

By looking carefully at the role-definitions we have chosen, we begin to have a truly fresh sense of new possibilities available, and a lot more air to breathe.

Physicians and nurses particularly get caught up in rigid role-definitions. In large part, this is due to the strong expectations of them from their patients. These rigid role-definitions contribute significantly to the stress and wear a medical staff may feel.

Process (for physicians and nurses)

Sit down and write out your description of your role as you see it. Physicians then write their description of nurses' role. Nurses then write their descriptions of physicians' role. Also, describe the role of the patient.

Now, form small groups and share your images and descriptions with one another. Notice similarities and differences. Notice what you expect from one another. Notice how you do/do not receive from the other just what you expect. For example: Doctors who see nurses as being warm and friendly, will experience more warm and friendly nurses in their day. And so on, with other expectations.

An example of a response may be similar to the following.

Nurse
How do you define your role?

> "My role is to give, help, be understanding. I'm not supposed to become angry, feel that I don't like a patient, or that I ever become repulsed. Of course, I do, sometimes. I feel I must seem cheerful, warm, and listen to whatever the physician tells me to do."

What are the rewards of this role for you?

> "There are many rewards for me. I feel good about myself. I feel like I'm helping and doing something really important. I learn about many people too. I've seen many people under real stress. I think I've grown stronger."

What is the main problem of this role for you?

> "It's hard to have to give so much all the time. Also, there is the friction with the physicians. I don't always want to listen to them. They can be obnoxious at times. It's as if we have no right to our own feelings or opinions."

Doctor
How do you define your role?

> "It's simple. I'm in charge of the patient and if anything goes wrong, it's because of me. There's a tremendous amount of responsibility here. I have to be strong, confident, and in charge all the time. This is what others expect of me. And they have a right to expect it. What kind of feeling would I create if I expressed doubt to a patient? It would be detrimental to the progress of the case."

What about when a patient is dying?

> "I personally do not view it that way. I do not feel that anyone is dying, until the very end. There is always something you can do.

We have to try everything. If I thought about them as dying, well, what would my function be? It's pretty depressing."

What are the rewards of this role for you?

"Well, of course I enjoy my work. I respect myself, the role is prestigious too. I won't deny that I like that. It's important to me. I like being successful. All in all, I'm pleased with myself."

What is the main problem of this role for you?

"It's when someone dies or complains too much. I feel like a failure, like I've done something wrong. Of course a patient is always ready to blame you for every little thing that goes wrong. You have to get used to it. But it gets to me, sometimes.

"There are other pressures too. I work long hours. There is a lot of tension. I have a home located on my own island. I feel I've earned it. This helps a great deal. Others have other ways of relieving the tension."

Patient
How do you define your role?

"What do you mean, how do I define my role? This isn't a role. I'm sick and I don't know why this has happened to me. I'm in pain all the time and I need to be taken care of. I don't like the role. I feel helpless and at the mercy of others. It's hard, very hard. Nobody really understands how I'm feeling."

What are the rewards of this role for you?

"Rewards? What are you saying? Well, I get out of work, I guess (laughs a little). And I get a lot of extra attention and care. Not enough though. I'm really able to see now who does and who does not love me."

What is the main problem of this role for you?

"Nobody believes me. I'm all alone. I've lost a lot of self-respect. I feel weak and I feel helpless. I feel like I'm a drain on others."

It is extremely interesting to have various individuals define their roles as they see them. Within their role-descriptions, we see the inherent rewards and problems that will arise.

Usually we find that a nurse's role-description is more open-ended and includes more feeling, nurturing, and mothering aspects. Many physicians forbid this to themselves and their patients. Physicians often want to be in control of themselves, the patients, the nurses, and the illness. When they feel they are losing control, a great deal of anguish arises.

The patient's role is often described as a completely dependent, helpless, and needful position. This myth has been widely perpetrated. But patients love to describe themselves as victims, the physicians as heroic rescuers, and the nurses as idealized mothers. Hospitals are often set up to intensify this kind of fantasy by the roles which everyone in them plays. Is this the best way to bring about real healing? Is it only the patient who is ill, or the entire system?

It is extremely refreshing, enjoyable, and illuminating to take roles that are opposite to the ones we usually play. There is no better way of opening our eyes and relieving tension, than of stepping into the other's shoes. It is also a wonderful way to be able to accept the other more deeply. We can directly experience what he or she is going through. As we do this, we may begin to allow our stereotyped images of another to melt away. We may also begin to allow ourselves more freedom in the responses we make.

Process

Here is a delightful process for physicians and nurses that will help each better understand and relate to the other. (This process can also be used by members of a family with a sick patient, as well as others.)

The scene is a hospital room. There are three players, the physician, nurse, and patient. A physician will play the roles of nurse or patient. A nurse will play the role of the physician or patient. A patient will play the roles of the doctor or nurse.

In this particular scene, *the physician* gives specific orders for a treatment plan to the nurse. *The nurse* has his or her own ideas about the treatment plan and is trying to express them to the physician. *The physician* is totally uninterested in the nurse's views. *The patient* wants to find out what is going on, and no one wants to tell him or her. The patient is viewed as a general nuisance.

Play around with the scenario. Adjust it any way you like. Play out the scene fully and then discuss it. See what feelings and insights come up for you. Create other suitable scenarios, which are relevant and familiar to you. Create scenes that will depict the kinds of problems and personalities that are difficult for you. Take another person's part in it. Take turns in playing all the roles. After it is over, notice what new understandings, perceptions, and possibilities arose.

An incredible amount of our misunderstandings and lack of communication come about through being glued to a particular role we live in. Unglue yourself a little. See if you can begin to separate yourself from the role-definition you have been living in. Our communication, perceptions, and responses are *constantly* being affected by the role we are living in.

Process

This process will help us distinguish the effects upon us and others of the particular role we are enacting. Take a partner. (There will be two parties, A and B.)

A, *pick a role you are comfortable with.* (Choose one that includes a certain amount of intimacy with *B*.) Now, tell B that he or she has a serious illness. B, respond. A, listen to B's response through the filter of your role.

A, *pick a role that is more distant* (possibly a professional role). Now, tell B the same news as before. B, respond again. A, listen to B's response through the filter of this role.

A, *pick a role you are uncomfortable with.* Now, tell B the same news as before. B, respond again. A, listen to B's response through the filter of this role. B, notice how your experiences and responses changed in all three conditions above. Discuss this fully with A.

Now, reverse roles, and do it all again.

When one becomes cast in the role of a patient, one is automatically alienated from one's own treatment process. Patients are no longer persons. Now, they have a specific function to fulfill. They become a part of a larger system.

This kind of system is often detrimental to the trust, openness, and well-being for all of the members. Despite their sense of power, physicians often feel lonely, anxious, and unloved. Despite their sense of goodness, nurses often experience the burden of their own unexpressed emotion and their own unexpressed need for love.

Stereotyped behaviors are demanded from everyone. This is difficult to live with on an on-going basis when we constantly are dealing with matters of life and death. The build-up of underlying stress can be unbearable.

Role-definitions are able to be loosened, opened, changed, and freshened. The best way to do this is to actually play out different kinds of scenes and to take roles that are different from the ones you are used to. Or, take the role you normally play and play it differently, as another kind of physician might.

We constantly need to stretch our horizons. If we do not expand and grow, we begin to atrophy. Nothing can stay the same forever. We are all living beings, and to live means to change.

Process

This is to explore ways of relating with patients. Following are two scenes described, for two kinds of physicians and patients. Take turns playing the various roles. Here, a third party, an observer, is required. This individual will have a list of questions (following the two scenes), and will intervene in the scene between the doctor and patient at an appropriate moment to ask the questions.

Physician A

> You have just learned definitely that this patient has an incurable carcinoma. Only palliative treatment is possible now. The patient has a life expectancy of three to six months.

> You are an authoritative physician and are used to directing the course of a patient's treatment without much discussion with the patient or family. However, you are kind and caring, and patients feel a sense of security with you.

> You are disturbed by the incorrect diagnosis and treatment this patient has received in the past. But nothing can be done about it now.

Patient A

You have been feeling ill for some time now (about six months).
You have been going to various physicians and have received
different impressions of what has been wrong. Nobody has been
absolutely clear with you about your illness.

Now you are experiencing increasing back pains, dizziness, and
faintness. You are frightened, tired, and want to get an answer at
any cost. All along you felt that the treatments you received were
not suitable, but you accepted the physician's opinion and did
nothing further. Now, you have made up your mind that you will
get to the truth of this situation.

Play this out together.

Physician B

You have just learned that this patient has an incurable carci-
noma, with a life expectancy of three to six months. Only
palliative treatment is possible now.

You are a warm, caring physician who is very emphatic and able
to relate to the patient's entire life situation. You are willing to
reflect back to the patient the truth of the situation as you see and
feel it to be. In fact, you feel it is very important to tell the truth as
much as you can.

Patient B

You have been growing progressively weaker for the past three
months, but have been feeling generally unwell for over six
months now. You do not like being sick and have never really
been sick in the past. You think of yourself as a strong person
with many ideas of your own.

You find this weakness to be tremendously annoying, but cannot
even imagine that you could ever become seriously ill. Other
physicians you have seen have given you mild treatments of
various kinds and have said your situation was not serious at all.

Now, you have fainted at work and are forced to consult with
Physician B.

Play this out together.

In the middle of the interactions already described, the observer comes in and says the following statements. The person he or she says them to, repeats and completes them.

The observer says the following statements to the physician, who has the patient complete them.

What I am feeling right now is _____.
What I want from you is _____.
What I want for you is _____.
If I were in your place, what I would now feel is _____.

When the physician finds that the patient is troubled, the observer intervenes with some other questions.

What is it you want right now? _____.
What do you believe that this behavior is doing for you? _____
What are you imagining is going to happen to you? _____
What is happening to you right now? _____

The observer is to allow the communication between the physician and the patient to continue for a while. Then the observer has the physician say the following to the patient.

Physician (to patient): I love you. I'll miss you.
Patient (to physician): I need you. I'm scared.

How does this make both of you feel? What are the effects of these statements that are out of the usually defined roles? Experiment with this.

Some have found that making these statements has entirely altered the climate and opened up brand new ways of being with one another. How do they affect you? Can you find some way to incorporate this in your relationship with those who are ill?

Sometimes the things we are most afraid of saying or doing, are the things which will bring the greatest help, clarity, and certainty. If we do not experiment, we can never be sure.

chapter seven
The Family

When illness comes the entire family network starts hurting. Everyone in it becomes sensitized and in greater need of attention and care. However, the family is often pushed aside. Many times the family is viewed as an annoyance, rather than as an ally and valuable aid in the patient's care.

Physicians and nurses become possessive of their patients. The patient now belongs to them. Decisions about the patient are now in their keeping. They may wish to protect a patient from some imagined problem with a family member. Loyalty to the patient develops and this loyalty may include wanting to keep some family member away.

A kind of rivalry with the family can begin. Physicians and nurses may begin to view the family as an adversary and the family can begin to feel afraid, as though their loved one is being taken away from them. They may feel as if they are being replaced in the patient's affections. Lines of dependence are shifting. A great deal of anxiety can get stirred up.

A medical staff may argue that a family member is beginning to demand too much of their time and attention. They may feel as if they inadvertently are getting caught up in the family network itself, because they are. No matter how distant they may wish to be, just their presence at this vital juncture makes them a temporary part of the family system, at least in the family's eyes. This may become difficult to handle, but once a physician (or nurse) is aware of this fact, he or she can then proceed with greater sensitivity and tact.

Some staff resent too much involvement with the family. They would rather devote their time to the patient. However, this feeling changes when we see that the patient and his or her family are inextricably interconnected. When you touch one part, the other feels it. The feelings, needs, and behaviors of the family members will inevitably have an effect upon the course of the patient's illness, perhaps even upon his or her desire to live. The whole picture, the whole constellation, must be attended to. In order to do this effectively, it is very valuable to understand the kind of dynamics that are going on in the family.

What are the family members experiencing? Some family members may not even be aware of it themselves. Often, there is simply a blanket sense of anxiety and sadness. Sometimes a family member becomes intrusive and demanding. This is just his or her way of reaching out for the help and support he or she needs. Or, sometimes a family member may be expressing the unconscious feelings of the patient him- or herself.

> *My sister is very ill; she's dying. It's not just her, it's me too. I'm also very ill and dying. I'm also facing all the fears and pain my sister is feeling. I look at her and I feel sick too. I need help too. I feel frightened.*
> *... Well, yes, now I just have to be extra strong, extra giving. I have to be understanding of her, no matter what she says to me. I was never understanding of her before. I'm trying my best. There's just nobody here being understanding of me.*
>
> Annette

This can be a very difficult situation for some family members. There is a strong expectation that the family member will love, support, and give to the patient in ways he or she was never able to before. Very little recognition is given to what the person, the family member, is feeling. All the attention is now turned to the patient. The patient now seems to be getting all of the love and care, which in itself can create a lot of jealousy and be difficult to bear.

> *My brother can't come to see me anymore. He came in the beginning, but where is he now? He's out on the streets alone, walking. I know it. I feel*

it. He can't give me all that love. He's hurting too much himself right now. I just wish I could see him so I could tell him I really understand.

Andrea, a seventeen-year-old girl dying of leukemia

It is unusual for a patient to have this much empathy and understanding. Instead, there is usually an implicit demand by the patient that the other family members come through for him or her. This expectation exists not only in the patient, but in the other family members as well. It is impossible not to be affected by it.

But a family member may not be able to come through for many reasons. There may have been a difficult or ambivalent relationship here in the past. Now suddenly this person is being called upon to be so loving. This is love that he or she just may not feel. Still, this pressure to love exists not only within him- or herself, but in the general family structure as well. If he or she does not comply with it, not only is there guilt within, but he or she may risk censure from the entire family as well. It is very important and helpful to bring this particular dynamic to light. Once it is brought out and discussed, a great deal of pressure may subside.

EXPRESSING GUILT

Anything that helps dissolve the pressure of guilt is an important adjunct to health. Guilt is both lethal and powerful in the family during a time of illness and loss. (Guilt in itself can be considered to be a form of terminal illness that constantly erodes the quality of our lives.) Unfortunately, much of the interaction between family members during a time of illness may stem largely from guilt.

There is the guilt that other family members are healthy, while this member is ill. A family member may be feeling that the patient is now ill because he or she did not love him or her enough, or give to the patient adequately in the past. Old difficulties in the relationship will now come up to be resolved. This in itself may be quite hard to handle.

The guilt does not go all in one direction. Patients may be feeling extremely guilty too. They may be feeling helpless, worthless, and unable to contribute to others. Many patients start to feel as if they have become a drain upon the entire family. Some express the wish that they were dead, rather than by laying there hurting others.

All interaction that arises from guilt inevitably produces discomfort. It does not ever provide the kind of satisfaction and comfort we are truly in need of.

By opening the way for an individual (or family) to become aware of, accept, and even express his or her feelings, a medical staff member can help a great deal, as the person will not feel so apart and alone. He or she will see that these feelings are natural, shared by others, and that they can become resolved. This in itself is very healing.

Sometimes it is possible to work more deeply with a family or patient. Sometimes a situation may require it. In that event, here is a wonderful process for helping a family deal with guilt. The basic principles of this process may also be applied in a variety of ways.

Process

What have you not yet done for the patient that you feel you really *should* do? Write it down. Make a list. Now, write down, what you think *the patient* would like you to do. Write down what *you* would really like to do. Notice the differences and similarities in your lists.

What has the patient not yet done for *you*, that you still want him or her to do? Write it down. Make a list. Can you ask the patient for what you want? Can you do for the patient what has to be done? Do you want to? What is getting in the way?

It is now tremendously helpful to discuss this all openly with the patient. Are you willing to try?

It is also very helpful to make a list of all the things you *have* done for the patient. Write down all the patient *has* done for you. Share this with the patient too. It is time to get accounts all settled.

This process can also be done by a patient, who is experiencing guilt with a given family member. The most helpful part, of course, is opening all of this up for discussion with one another. When it is possible to freely share these feelings, tremendous relief and renewal is possible. It is also much easier to do what yet remains to be done, and to let go of what we are unable to do. (We may often be surprised to discover that the patient did not want that anyway.) In this way, we get a reprieve from ourselves and each other, while clearing up all that is unessential away.

EXPRESSING ANGER AND RESENTMENT

While guilt may be common in some cases, there may be fury and unexpressed resentment going on in others. In fact, a patient's entire illness may have been generated by his or her anger and the inability to express it directly.

It is not at all unusual to see a family in which there has been a great deal of unresolved anger and animosity. In a situation of this type, a family member can become rather frightened by the illness of the patient. A family member may feel that he or she has somehow hurt the patient, even caused the patient to be ill. Family members can become overly protective and worried about every little thing that goes on. They will not leave the hospital. They will not leave the patient alone. There may be considerable overcompensation taking place.

It feels unacceptable to us to express angry feelings or personal hurts to someone when he or she is ill. (This is why many people enjoy becoming ill.) There is the implicit feeling that the patient is suffering enough already and that he or she could not possibly take anything more. Also, we may be feeling that we cannot expect anything more from the patient. (This feeling alone can cause a great deal of anger and hurt.)

We usually react by bottling up our feelings and trying to hide how upset we are. This gives less and less reality to the relationship, bringing only distance between us and the patient. The patient senses this happening and starts to feel even more alone, as if he or she has nothing to hold onto anymore.

> *I feel like a murderer. Everytime I look into her eyes, I feel like I did it. I've always just hated her guts. Now I'm scared. Does she know it? Did I do this to her somehow?*
>
> Johnathan

This kind of reaction in a family member may develop into guilt later on. Johnathan may start punishing himself in various ways after the death of this patient, having no idea at all why this is happening. Or, he may begin to deny any anger and start viewing her as a "saint." Then he will view himself as the bad one.

It is good and healthy to express, to allow, and to accept anger. Family members (especially children), must be helped to see that feelings do not kill another and that one person's illness is *never* created by the next. (Even if we wished someone dead a thousand times, our wishes do not make them die. These wishes only fill *us* with torment.)

BLAME

Family members and friends, who are filled with unacknowledged anger and self-blame, often project these feelings onto the staff. They are constantly finding fault with everyone else. Unfortunately, this is a familiar occurrence on the hospital floor. Such an individual simply needs to be helped to acknowledge his or her own feelings of inadequacy and guilt.

In such a case, a doctor or nurse may help individuals such as these greatly simply by telling them that they are not to blame for what is going on. It is surprising how much this may calm these individuals. Of course, they may need to hear it over and over. They may need to realize, too, that they are not in control of this patient's life, not of his or her sickness or wellness. They must be brought to understand that after all, they are only two travellers going along the same road together. No matter how much they love their brother or sister, give to him or her, and want to help him or her, ultimately each person has to answer for his or her own life.

In this connection it is also very important for the medical staff to realize that the blame that this individual is putting on them, is only a reflection of the individual's bad feelings about him- or herself. A medical staff can best react to this instance by helping this person see and accept what is going on within; to help make the person feel better about him- or herself somehow.

The greatest gift we have to give to one another is self-awareness and self-acceptance. We cannot let another love us if we are busy hating ourselves. By reflecting and acknowledging an individual's feelings, we give him or her both self-awareness and our acceptance, which helps the individual accept him- or herself.

How can this be accomplished? A simple statement like the following can work wonders. "You must be feeling very worried about your brother. Perhaps you feel you have not yet done all you could do? Perhaps you are angry with yourself?"

Sometimes this kind of opening will help individuals express other feelings as well to you. Listen, acknowledge, and accept their feelings. This will relieve them of guilt and self-blame. (It is not necessary to offer directives of any kind.) Simply by virtue of individuals being able to see that others understand and accept them, they will be helped to find their own way.

We all share the same feelings and thoughts. In truth, nothing is strange or unusual. Each person's reaction is your reaction too. Nobody is all alone.

MANIPULATION AND CONTROL

Another form of unexpressed, unacknowledged anger that may be taking place in a family during illness, is that of manipulation and control. There is no one as powerful as a sick person. The weaker and sicker we are, the more we create feelings of guilt and obligation in those around us, the more others feel they must monitor their feelings. The more we can get, the more we want! What a tremendous trap this can be!

This kind of power is most difficult to deal with (both for families and for a medical staff) because it is covert, subtle, and goes unrecognized for long periods of time. It does not go unfelt though. It works intently, whether we know it or not.

Certain patients, certain family members use their illnesses to get all they can get. Their illnesses become a sudden opportunity for them to make all kinds of claims upon others, claims they may have felt they had no right to before. This kind of domination can be overpowering. Family members need protection too.

Process

What do you feel you would be entitled to if you got sick that you are not entitled to now? What are you willing to give another, because they are sick, that you would not give them regularly? If you knew you only had a short while to live, what would you then be able to give to yourself that you are not able to give now? Why can't you give it to yourself now?

Write the answers down. Discuss them with someone else. Make them as specific as possible.

A patient may have been needy and hungry for a very long time. Now, all of a sudden, the illness serves to let it all loose. The patient may suddenly feel that he or she has a right to now have all needs met. And fast! Or else!

Family members can become overcome by the demands and so-called needs of a tyrannical patient. Although this is a delicate matter, it should be looked at carefully.

A particular patient may be deriving so many benefits and pleasures out of the role of being sick that he or she can become unconsciously determined not to get well again. Why should he or she? The patient may be enjoying his or her illness to its maximum!

It is also possible that a family member is enjoying the patient's sickness too. (No illness can go on for a really long time without the cooperation and support of others.) Be careful, become aware. Perhaps the illness is making the healthy family member feel quite important now, as suddenly he or she is needed.

The family member may also be feeling rather powerful. At last he or she is stronger than the patient! Perhaps the family member has some new-founded power over the patient. Or, the illness might bring a sense of security to someone in the family. Now the member knows that the patient won't go away. Other family members can become subtly afraid of the patient's recovery. They may be so much enjoying this newly founded intimacy.

The entire matter is quite complex and it is necessary to be aware of all the components. These may be having a strong effect upon the course of recovery.

Some patients become sick in order to "get back," to make someone else in the family pay. They may be saying implicitly, "Now you have to take care of me, whether you like it or not. You didn't love me enough before. You just have to love me now." The price for this kind of love is sickness and pain. Some pay it willingly. They are pleading, "I'll stay helpless and weak if only you will love me."

What price do you feel *you* have to pay for the love and care you are receiving? What price are others paying, in order to feel loved by you?

Not too many family members are strong enough to remain unmoved by the needs and demands of this kind of tyranny. Most begin to comply, and begin to feel trapped. They are not trapped by the patient really, but by their own feelings of guilt and fear, as well as by their confusion about what is going on.

In this case, complying with the demands of the patient can only make matters worse and worse. When we give out of compulsion, the need of the person to whom we are giving only intensifies. What we are giving does not satisfy and the person may seem insatiable.

As the person's insatiability grows, our own sense of inadequacy deepens. Nothing we give will ever be enough! The more we give in such a manner, the unhappier we all become. All of this can become a case of psychic blackmail.

How do we extricate ourselves and the other from this bind which we fall in? How do we determine what is reasonable, how much we can give with comfort and ease? How do we learn to say *enough* in all good conscience, feeling secure in the knowledge that we have really done our humanly best? This in itself is a very good feeling. When we feel this way it does not matter how the other one receives our gift.

First of all, in order to extricate ourselves from this bind, it is necessary to understand that if we are giving *at our own expense* (if we are suffering as a result of what we are giving), then it is *not* true giving at all, and will only backfire on both parties. If we are giving out of fear, sadness, or desperation then that is exactly what our gift will contain: fear, sadness, and desperation. All we have to give, all we ever give to anyone is our own state of being. The rest is superfluous. It is always only ourselves that we are giving. If we come to a bedside grim, exhausted, and filled with a sense of obligation, then we are only giving poison. Better to stay home and lie in the sun. Better for both of you. The patient does not need to feel your resentment. It will only make him or her feel worse; smaller, sadder.

However, this resentment will not be present when you can say *no* comfortably, when you can listen to your own inner rhythm, find your own balance, and determine what you can comfortably give. Then give it gladly and you will feel wonderful. If the person wants more, you will be able to refuse them and to refuse them still feeling good. Most people can't do this at all.

Who have you refused lately? How did you feel? When do you plan to do it again?

Most of us get angry with others for wanting things from us because we feel we cannot say *no* to them. We feel we must give whatever is requested, no matter how outlandish, no matter whether or not we have it to give.

Process

Now we will examine this entire matter more closely. First, look at yourself. How much do you feel you must give to another? (Pick an important person in your life and assess him or her. Pick someone less important to you and again assess him or her.)

What is your cut off point? What would you absolutely *not* do, or give up, for the person? What kind of giving is easiest for you? What do you like to give most? Why? What kind of giving makes you feel replenished? What kind of giving makes you feel ill? (Try to remember some situations where this happened.) Who do you most like to give to? Why?

Write all of this down and share it with another if possible.

In order to go one step further, you will need a partner. One person is A, the other B.

A, ask B for something. B, can you give it? Do you want to? A, ask B for more. And more. And more. And more. (A, notice what you are asking for) Keep this going. A, see how much you are able to ask for and how much you feel you are entitled to receive.

B, see how much you are able to give (and willing). B, see when you can say *no*. How do you feel when you say it? What do you want to do to A now?

Next reverse roles. Both partners are to discuss their feelings and what they saw about themselves.

It is important to see what is prompting our giving. Sometimes we have fantasies and feelings about what the patient is going through. We are then giving to the patient to allay our own fantasies and fears. It may have nothing at all to do with what he or she wants, or is going through.

Please take some time and check this out.

Process

Imagine what the patient is now going through. Put yourself in his or her shoes and fantasize what it is like to actually be the patient. Write about it, draw it, discuss it. What do you think is going to happen to the patient? How do you want to stop this from happening?

Now, ask the person about *his* or *her* experience. How does it compare with your fantasies?

It can also be helpful to gather concrete, practical information about what "exactly" is taking place from the medical staff. How does this compare with your fantasies?

Sometimes we become so identified with a member of our family, that we become confused about our differing responses and needs. We may have no real idea of what *that* person is wanting. It may be impossible to realize even that *that* person is different from ourselves. Sometimes we do not even see that we are really two separate people. (This phenomenon is particularly obvious when at the death of one family member, the other becomes suicidal.)

In these kinds of cases, it is good to focus upon the ways in which the family member is different from the patient. What are their separate likes and goals?

DISTINCTIONS AND CLARIFICATIONS

Process

If you were in _____'s shoes right now, what would *you* be wanting? Do *you* want this now? What do you feel that _____ is needing now? Can you find out directly from _____ what he or she really needs and wants?

So many of us are busy giving to the other that which *we* ourselves truly want to receive. We can't give it to ourselves, but we can give it to another. Then we wait to get it back from him or her. We may end up waiting a very long time.

When we can give to ourselves directly, it is so much easier to give to the next. It is hard to give truly when we feel empty. When we give while feeling empty, the other may feel he or she is robbing us. But it is entirely natural to share ourselves with another, when we are feeling full.

> *Make yourself*
> *Like the autumn lake,*
> *Full of water*
>
> Old Zen saying

What do *you* want at this very moment? Are you able, willing, to give it to yourself?

When we are with the sick or dying, we are giving them more than our presence, we are giving them their presence, too. Everything we do or feel has an effect upon them. Even the way we view another will have an effect upon how they feel.

When we see someone as sick, weak, and helpless, that is exactly how he or she begins to feel around us. The more sick the patient seems to us, the worse he or she begins to feel. Our very perception and image of him or her begins to affect his or her way of responding.

Process

Stop for a moment, and try to see the person you are with as beautiful. Focus upon their good points and beauty. Now watch and see how they respond to you.

We must always be conscious of the kind of image we are perpetuating with a given person, particularly with someone who is ill. How do you see this particular patient? Stop for a moment, and take notice of it.

Process

Write down a description of the person as you see him or her.
List whatever adjectives come to your mind about the patient. Draw
a picture of him or her. Are you focusing upon the patient's weakness? Are you in touch with his or her strengths and abilities? If the
person is dying, are you viewing him or her as a "goner," or as
someone about to embark upon an exciting journey?

Your view of the other is always being communicated to him or
her, whether you want it to be or not. Are you looking at the patient
with pity and disgust? Can you look through the eyes of admiration?

Examine your reactions closely. You can alter your images. How
you perceive the patient is a matter of your choice. You can choose to
see and relate to his or her courage, life, and ability to love, rather
than to the parts of the individual that are failing. This choice is
always in your keeping.

What do you relate to in yourself?

Process

Find five beautiful things about the patient, just exactly as he or
she is now. Write them down. Share them with the patient.

Find five beautiful things about yourself, just exactly as you are
now. Write them down. Share them with the patient.

Find five positive things about the situation you both are
presently in. Write them down. Share them with the patient.

A sick individual will find it harder to become well when those
around him or her are people who view him or her with dread and
gloom. By relating primarily to the part of the person that is sick and
ailing, we may be suppressing actual recovery. We may be suppressing the part in the individual that is strong, vital, and well. This
part exists within every one of us.

The more attention you give one aspect, the more it blossoms
under your eyes. When patients start to become well again, it is
because they become in touch with their natural desire to live and be
well. Just like sap in the trees, this desire, this natural healing force,
can rise in each one of us. By relating to that which is well and
positive, you are encouraging this to flow.

We may have been feeling that to be a good family member, to really love the other, meant to do whatever the patient wanted us to do. This kind of loving causes dependency, which is not the same feeling as love. We also may have been feeling that telling ourselves that the person is sick and weak is our way of understanding the individual, of giving him or her leeway. This is only true to a point.

True love means relating to the strong parts. True love strengthens, enables, sets free. Dependency cuts a person down. It weakens and saddens and makes you feel wobbly.

True love respects another person's choices. Dependency holds a person too close. There is a necessary time for weaning, the child from the mother; the mother from the child.

The best way to know if we are really loving one another is to look at the effects our behavior is having upon the individual. When a person is truly loved, he or she will blossom. It cannot be any other way. Are we giving in order to hold the individual, or in order to set him or her free?

When we are truly loving another, we also feel loved and complete. There is nothing the person has to do particularly to earn or to deserve our love. We love the person just because he or she is. We love the individual and our love makes *us* happy. This is what makes us happy, not what we are given in return.

Please stop and look at yourself for a moment.

What makes you feel most loved?
When do you really feel loved and cared for?
When do you feel unloved and ignored?
How are you helped to feel your strongest?

The deepest act of love is to help others to love themselves, admire themselves, to feel good and worthy. This is a way of extending an invitation to others to live and be well.

> *Real love leaves no traces,*
> *It touches and departs,*
> *Just like an angel.*
>
> Eshin

chapter eight
Communication
With the Family

Many difficulties arise in communication between the family and the medical staff. This chapter is dedicated to practical ways in which this can be best handled for both parties.

Families (and patients) place physicians on a pedestal and many physicians like to stay there. It may feel nice up there on the pedestal, but the air is rarified and it can become difficult to get through to those on the ground. Sometimes the pedestal becomes wobbly and physicians (or nurses) begin to feel separate and away from the crowd.

Generally, physicians are trained to view the patient impersonally. This kind of distancing has important components for the physician, helping him or her to maintain necessary objectivity. However, there are dangers too. The physician can also become distanced from him- or herself and from the feelings he or she is experiencing. This distancing, or suppression of feelings, can take a real toll in the physician's (or nurse's) life. Many experience considerable stress that may be directly related to this position of impersonality. They have chosen a particular way of relating with the patient that may not sufficiently include recognition and expression of their own feelings and needs.

Generally, there are three basic role patterns through which medical staff relate to patients.

1. *Leader* In this pattern, the physician (or nurse) becomes a role model for the family and portrays the behavior he or she may feel it is presently in need of; strength, structure, authority. He or she is generally in command of the situation, and may even seem impervious to feelings of sadness, love, and doubt. While this role offers security to the family, it may also increase the members' feelings of dependency and helplessness.

2. *Mirror* In this pattern, the physician (or nurse) does not enter or intervene directly with the family unit. Instead, he or she remains a neutral observer, offering clarity and objective concern. The focus here is *not* upon the relationship, but upon the awareness and understanding that his or her presence facilitates.

While this position relates to the patient's strength, in this kind of situation a patient may sometimes feel that the physician or nurse lacks kindness and warmth.

3. *Human* Here the physician (or nurse) plays no particular role at all. He or she simply shares his or her humanity with the family through expressing personal feelings and neither seeks nor refuses personal involvement.

In this case, the experience of the patient is that of being with a full person who is really there for him or her. This may be rather frightening to some patients who wish the support of a strong authority figure. For others, this kind of relating offers maximal courage and strength.

It is an art in itself to know which role position is called for, at which times, and with which particular patient. Generally, a physician or nurse assumes one of these role patterns on a more or less consistent basis. However, it is enriching to see that these roles are not immutable. We tend to wear only one garment and feel we can never take it off. However, these particular role garments are interchangeable. It is necessary to develop flexibility and be able to find ways to wear all three.

In order to do this successfully, we must become aware of the patients we deal with and the ways in which they differ. We must also become more fully aware of our own responses to different patients.

Naturally, some patients (and families) are more difficult than others for us to deal with. Usually, we handle these cases in an automatic manner, trying our best to keep our distance. It is most instructive to stop for a moment and look closely at the patients who are hard for you to handle. It's not necessarily that *they* are most difficult. It's that they are giving *you* a difficult time. Something about this particular patient stimulates some disturbance in you. (Actually, they are doing you a service. Now you have the opportunity to learn something more about *you*).

Rather than focus on the faults of the patients, it is more useful to focus on the reaction that is going on inside of you. You cannot change their shortcomings, but you *can* alter what *you* feel. Withdrawing from a patient (in one way or another) really does nothing at all; not for you or for the patient. Sooner or later they will return once again. Until we deal fully with a person or relationship that is hard for us, it will come back to us over and over to be fully understood. This is unavoidable.

Process

Look at the patients (or families) that are disturbing you. What specifically about them is hard to take? How does their responding make you feel about yourself? What are they asking from you that you may or may not want to give them?

Now, right at this moment, try seeing *these* patients or families in a different way. Actively find one sympathetic point or quality about them. Find something within yourself that you can truly give to them. What is it? Give it, please. Let them say thank you, if they want to.

Do this same process with patients (or families) that are particularly congenial for you. Why exactly are you so comfortable? What are they giving to you?

It is very useful to do this process right on the spot when you find yourself in a specific interaction that is giving you trouble. In order to be able to use it on the spot, with ease, you must practice it alone by yourself and acquire familiarity with your personal process.

To prepare yourself to use this technique, first make a list for yourself of the kinds of patients who are difficult for you. Then, make a list of the kinds of patient and family situations you have difficulty with.

When we communicate with others, ultimately it is only with some part of ourselves. Each person with whom we are communicating can be thought of as a mirror in which we see our own beauty or our own flaws. What we cannot accept in others, is a part we have rejected within ourselves. (Otherwise this quality would just leave us neutral.)

So now, look again at this difficult patient and say the following to yourself.

1. "What is it about this patient I am not willing to accept in myself?"
2. Try supporting the person you dislike the most.
3. Identify with the person you feel the most distant from.
4. Look carefully at your *own* reactions.
5. Say to yourself, "This is a part of me too."

By accepting everybody we come into contact with, ultimately we are learning how to love and accept ourselves too. Really, who can ever exhibit behavior that one is not somehow capable of?

Process

Now we will go more deeply into a difficult interaction, in order to know it in greater depth.

This is a role-playing process. Three people are needed: The physician (or nurse); the patient; and the observer: A, B, and C.

1. Physician (or nurse) will describe a patient (family) or situation that he or she consistently has had difficulty with.
2. Together the physician (or nurse) and the patient will create and play out the difficult situation, just as it would go on in life.
3. The observer will watch and interject questions.

As the scene proceeds, the observer interrupts in the middle, with statements and questions out loud. The physician repeats them after the observer and completes them on the spot. The patient responds to the physician any way he or she likes. Then, the observer does it again and the patient repeats the statements and completes them. The physician responds to the patient any way he or she likes. The statements and questions the observer asks follow.

1. What I am feeling right now is _____.
2. What I want from you right now is _____.
3. What I want *for* you right now is _____.
4. If I were in _____ place right now I would feel _____.

If the patient is persistent and difficult, the physician asks the following.

1. What do you believe this behavior is doing for you?

Now, the observer is to pause and have the physician say the following to the patient. "I'm sorry about your situation. I care about you and I will miss you." The patient is to respond to the physician by saying, "Please be kind to me because I'm afraid, and I very much need you."

Continue the scene now after these interventions. How is the communication affected? How has the atmosphere changed? How has your behavior altered? Experiment with this for a while, then notice what other possibilities became available to you after these interventions. Were you willing to try them? Were you aware of them while they were going on? Would you be willing to try them out in the future?

Now, reverse roles. Someone else be the physician, the patient, and the observer. Proceed same as before.

When we become able to expand our collection of behaviors, we become more available both to our patients and to one another. Just by being aware that you have many options, your feelings of stress will be diminished. When you actually become able to experiment with these various options, then you will create an atmosphere in which difficult problems easily become resolved.

Sometimes it is not a particular patient, but an entire family configuration that is giving us trouble. One member may be attempting to receive the support of the physician or nurse in collusion against the next. Perhaps the member may ask the physician or nurse not to tell another person (the patient maybe) what exactly is going on. Immediately, a bind is being created for the physician or the nurse, as loyalties are being questioned.

In some families there is a covert agreement among members to keep the patient in the dark. This may go under the guise of telling the physician or nurse that the patient is weak and cannot handle the situation emotionally. In a case like this, stop for a moment and look at the emotional condition of the family member who is telling you that. This person may be trying to make the physician or nurse a pawn in their relationship with the patient.

Of course, the optimal situation for the physician or nurse is when he or she is very clear about his or her own position and able to state it clearly to the family. Some physicians have refused to work with certain patients when the family has insisted that they may not tell the patient the truth. This is a highly personal decision on the part of the physician. Usually the matter is not quite so clear-cut. Often there are strains and binds that the physician and nurse are subjected to daily that they themselves are unaware of.

Process

This process is for the purpose of clarifying what is going on, to the family, to the patient, and to the staff. Again, we turn to a role-playing process, where individuals may assume different parts. (It is helpful to do the process in two ways: first take a role different from the one you normally play, then play the one you normally play. It is also valuable to play out your role as you usually do, and then hear the responses of others in the discussion that follows.)

Following are some suggested characters and situations. Naturally, these may be altered to suit your particular needs.

1. *Family Member* You consider yourself to be a strong, successful individual with excellent judgment. You are now determined to take over the course of your brother's illness. You are very close to your brother and have dominated him for a long while now. You are beginning to become frightened by the extent of his illness, and·have begun to fear that he might die. You feel extremely responsible for his well-being and for protecting him. You feel your brother is weak and overly sensitive. Above all else, you do not want him to know the full extent of his illness. Generally, you do not trust doctors and certainly do not wish to be replaced in the over-all care of your brother. As the physician speaks to you, you do not believe anything you are told. You feel that you know best.

2. *Patient*   You have been feeling very weak and sick for some-time now and have not yet felt that you are getting anywhere. Different physicians have told you different things and you do not trust them at all. However, you rather like this particular physician and very much want to listen to your physician and believe what you are told. Above all, you want to know definitively just what is going on.

3. *Doctor*   Your patient has advanced cancer. You have just made a definitive diagnosis. Now you wish to communicate the diagnosis to the patient and outline a treatment plan which you feel *may be* effective in this situation. You want to be open and honest, as this is your general style. Also, you are rather an authoritative physician who likes to take complete charge of your case. The patient's brother is driving you crazy.

There are many kinds of situations which will arise. Sometimes a physician must intervene on behalf of a patient. Sometimes a physician may want to intervene on a family member's part. Some-times a physician must deal with the hostility and fear of the other family members toward him- or herself or toward the patient.

In cases where patients are too weak to speak up for them-selves, the physician or nurse may assist by identifying with the patient, and speaking for him or her to the family. A comment like the following one may offer a great deal of help. "Right now Jane requires your support. You cannot make any more demands of her presently."

Here the physician or nurse is bringing the family's attention both to the reality of the situation and to their behavior in it. He or she may wish to intensify the family's awareness of their behavior and ask a question or two such as the following. "What is it you are wanting from Jane right now? What exactly do you feel your be-havior is doing for you?"

When there is a great deal of confusion and pain going on in the family and patient's interaction, it may be appropriate to suggest that the family themselves (and also the patient) begin to do some role-playing. They can each take various roles in the family, or, they can play the physician's role. Often this rather strong and sometimes startling intervention serves to loosen up, clarify, and brighten the atmosphere considerably.

Very often, most family members are suffering from a great deal of guilt. This fact should always be uppermost in the physician's and nurse's awareness. All kinds of difficult and offensive behavior can be directly traced to guilt. When you have a close relationship with the family, and see clearly that this is going on, a statement like the following can be of tremendous help. "No matter what you might have wanted to do for Jane up to now, you *did* whatever you were able. If you *could have* done more, you would have. Can you forgive yourself now, and just let it be?"

A remark like this is often startling to a patient (or a family member). When so much acceptance is offered from an authority figure, this in itself often helps to alleviate considerable guilt. Certainly, at the very least, it provides an entirely new way for the patient to view the situation. When family members or patients realize that you are not judging them harshly, they can then be kinder to themselves, too.

It is wonderful to overtly express any positive perceptions you have. We often assume that people know how we are feeling. When we have positive feelings, it is good to reinforce this by expressing them directly.

Stop and look at the way you are "viewing" the other from time to time. In some part of the other person, he or she is feeling it, too. What are your true feelings? What are your fantasies about the other person? Are you willing to express and share some part of the other individual? Are you willing to stop for a moment and see how the other might be viewing you? He or she may be afraid of you and may be feeling particularly needful of some warmth from you. Look at the other person with just this in mind; to see what it is he or she wants from you. Can you give it to the other person?

We fear this attitude is not "professional." Boundaries will be lost and our effectiveness will dissipate. However, just the opposite is true. When individuals feel truly seen, heard, and responded to, then the optimal interaction can take place.

Following is a summary of the main points of the chapter, so as to have them readily available for your continuing use.

Use Yourself   By experiencing and sharing your feelings (as they are happening) with the patient and family, you are creating an atmosphere which is optimal for all.

Role-Reversal   This is a wonderful means to open up your awareness of a situation and to find new possibilities for dealing with it. It allows you to see the world through the eyes and heart of another, and it allows the other to see the world through your eyes. Create scenes which depict your most difficult characters and situations, and play them out with partners.

Relieve Guilt   Most people are suffering greatly under self-imposed guilt and blame. A great deal of criticism directed at others comes directly from this source. Help the patient and family be relieved of this burden. Point out what can still be done realistically. Point out to the patient and family what has already been given. Help each person set the other free.

Real Giving   Real giving does not demand a great deal back in return, nor does it foster dependency. It is not based on sacrifice. It also helps another become strong and free.

> *Generosity means not possessing. Generosity is just a state of mind where one does not want to possess.*
>
> Chogyam Trungpa

> *Dried salmon*
> *received, and oranges*
> *given in return.*[1]
>
> Shiki

---

[1]From *Peonies Kana: Haiku by the Upasaka Shiki,* translated by Harold J. Isaacson. The Bhaisajaguru Series. Copyright © 1972 by Harold J. Isaacson. Used by permission of Theater Art Books, 153 Waverly Place, New York, NY 10014.

chapter nine

Understanding
and Handling Pain

What is it we expect when we are in despair and yet go to a man? Surely, a presence through whom we can feel that somehow there still is meaning.[1]

Buber

We take it for granted that pain is terrible and must be avoided at all costs. As soon as we start to feel some pain, even a minor discomfort, we look for pills and physicians; anything at all to suppress the pain. Sooner or later though, the pain returns. Why? We forget to ask the fundamental question, "What is this pain?"

Instead, we run blindly away from pain and don't stop to wonder just what it is that we are running away from. Is it possible to escape it? Is it necessary we should?

We must consider what this pain is exactly, and why it is in our lives *now*. Where is it coming from? Why is it coming to us? Is this pain necessary, perhaps even good?

Some feel that pain is a punishment, or perhaps a kind of teaching. But usually, we avoid the entire matter. It seems simpler to feel sorry for ourselves and seek comfort and ease. Although there is

[1] Excerpts from Martin Buber, *Between Man and Man*, copyright © 1965 by Macmillan Publishing Co. Used by permission of Macmillan Publishing Co., Inc., and Routledge & Kegan Paul, Ltd.

nothing wrong with comfort and ease, it never really handles the matter.

The Buddha has said that all life is suffering. What did he mean by this? This statement has been misunderstood many times. Many have thought it to be a negation of our lives, while just the opposite is true. This statement simply wants to point out that which obscures true living. By truly understanding the nature of suffering, we have the possibility of ending it. The Buddha considered himself a doctor with medicine for suffering. What kind of suffering was Buddha talking about? What does this have to do with the physical pain we experience during a time of illness?

There is only one pain, and it manifests itself in various ways. It can come physically, mentally, or emotionally. According to Buddha, all pain comes from desire. We long for something and cannot have it. Or, we can have it and then fear to lose it. When we do inevitably lose it, we suffer the *pain of loss and change*.

We are always longing and clinging. In the very midst of life, we long for more life. As we finish one meal, we are already dreaming of the next. This kind of suffering, the suffering of insatiable hunger is called the *pain of greed*. It is based on the feeling that we can never be full and satisfied.

Perhaps we are longing for conditions to be different. In the midst of illness, we long for health. We refuse to accept our condition at the moment. Somehow we are not able to accept each moment just as it is. We must change life, fix it, overpower it with our own expertise. We have so many ideas about how everything in life *should* be, but life itself doesn't really care about our particular plans. The pain of this attitude is called the *suffering of arrogance*.

The worst kind of pain is the pain which comes at random, suddenly, for no known reason. We cannot grasp what is happening. We do not know what the pain is signifying and feel it is senseless pain. All human beings require meaning. We need to grasp what is happening. Is it possible that we are going to die? This kind of pain is also called *anguish*.

What has all this to do with the intense physical pain that many feel during an illness? Some would suggest that there is really no difference between our physical pain, between our illness, and between the emotional and mental pain we go through.

There is only one pain because we are one. Looking at one aspect of our suffering, we are also inevitably looking at the next. All aspects are inextricably connected.

At the bedside of someone in physical pain, when we deal with the emotional, mental, or spiritual aspects, often the physical pain will startlingly subside. This is not unusual or surprising, but rather natural. When people have a strong emotional illness that is expressed that way, they are often very healthy physically. Or, when physical illness erupts, the emotional turbulence becomes suppressed.

When physical illness comes, we usually do not view it as part of a larger condition of distress. Instead, we focus on the physical symptoms, which may be only the tip of the iceberg. In order for real healing to come, the individual may have to make other changes in his or her total life.

There are constant bacteria, germs, and diseases within us. Suddenly, one day, they get the upper hand. At other times, they recede. Why?

Illness can come when we feel defeated and when we may not even want to live anymore. (When we are in love, there is not much time for illness). Or, some people become ill in order to tell themselves that it is time to make other changes in their lives. Each illness has its own story.

Process

Think of three times in your life when you felt particularly upset, sad, or defeated. How did you handle it? How did you express it? What happened to you physically? What happened to other parts of your life?

We usually view illness as an enemy, as something separate from ourselves that we must do battle with. We do not usually see the illness simply as an expression of our deeper selves. We seldom consider that the illness itself may be curing the patient. What is the real illness? What is the real cure?

We become sick because we act in sickening ways.

Louis Jourard

Modern medicine is based on the notion of battle. We battle germs and fight for life, but by removing the symptoms the true illness may be repressed. Inevitably though, it will have to return.

Cancer can be suppressed for many years and a person continues to live. But then it reappears. So, we must ask: Why this cancer *now*? What is going on in my total life? What is this cancer saying to me about all aspects of myself?

The usual experience is to feel that we are walking along beautifully one day and all of a sudden the pain and illness attack us from out of nowhere, which is not true. We have not been walking along beautifully. Something has been going wrong for a long time, but we have been overlooking it. We are afraid of change. We are afraid to notice the quality of our lives, moment to moment, day by day. We are all experts at brushing things under the carpet. Then the carpet begins to give away, because there is just too much mess. The corners begin to roll up. We feel as if we are coming unglued—and we are. This is not necessarily bad, it may just mean that it's time to clean under the carpet.

The pain and illness are now demanding that you pay attention to all that you left unattended before. You have no choice but to listen to what is going on inside. Are you willing to listen and to respond? (This is a very important question. Take it seriously by stopping for a moment to really consider it.)

Death can come from years of accumulated sorrow and hurt. Then, all of a sudden, it's too much anymore. Cancer can come from years of accumulated resentment, bitterness, and fear. Then, all of a sudden, it's too much anymore.

Your body rebels. You are also your body and you may have been pushing yourself for too long. Now your body is fed up with it. It is telling you to stop and listen! You could have listened, you could have noticed before, but we are not taught to live with respect for what we are feeling.

The first step out of this maze is to realize that this pain, this unrecognized aspect of ourselves, is now demanding to be listened to. When we learn how to listen and how to reply, we begin to live an entirely new life. Clearly, the pain and illness can become an opportunity for real growth and change. We are being asked to look at, hear, and accept other aspects of ourselves; to integrate ourselves in a new way.

Some people reject one aspect of themselves or another. Some reject their emotions, bodies, minds, or spirits. No matter whether we reject a part or not, sooner or later it must be attended to.

For example, if we are sad for too long and have not done enough crying, our bodies may begin to cry for us, through one illness or the next. If we feel that life is simply meaningless, our bodies will express this, by shriveling up and dying. If we have held onto difficult attitudes, our bodies will bear the burden of these. Whatever we feel or believe inevitably appears in our bodies.

Let us look at some of the attitudes we live with and take for granted as practical truths. Are these attitudes conducive to health? Or, are these attitudes themselves the very seeds of pain?

We believe that life is difficult, that we must suffer, struggle, and have a hard time of it. Many pride themselves on how much they struggle. Nature does not struggle. When spring comes, thousands of flowers just bloom naturally.

We believe life is full of pain and defeat. Fear is a constant companion. Disappointment is a usual feeling. We never question these beliefs. Our pain and illness become the testimony that this is so.

We do not allow ourselves too much beauty or pleasure. We drive ourselves relentlessly, as even our leisure is filled with competitive, aggressive pastimes. Is it any wonder we become so ill and racked with pain? In order to truly handle the illness, we must also handle our attitudes.

Process

Make a list of the fundamental attitudes you have about your life. How do these attitudes affect your daily living? What kind of toll do they take on you? How can you change them? What kind of health-giving attitudes could you replace them with?

When we are in pain, we want the nurse or the physician to take over and control our illness by giving us something to make us feel better. This attitude in itself is part of the original disease. We are relinquishing our part in the illness. We are denying the fact that it is up to us to stop and listen to the meaning of our illness and to find our own appropriate response. This does not suggest that we do not go to the physician or accept appropriate medication. It only suggests that the physician and the medicine are only one part of the treatment. We must do our part as well. We must listen to, accept, and understand our pain.

For many people the word *accept* has bad connotations. It implies being weak and giving in. Nothing can be further from the truth. Acceptance is a vital act, full of strength and courage. To accept means *to know* the pain, to let it in, and to become acquainted. To accept means to *make friends* with the moment, with your entire experience, and not fight it or push it away. What results is a welcoming attitude toward all of existence.

The value of accepting the pain is that suddenly it is not really pain anymore but just another part of our own being and very soon passes away. This attitude helps dissolve the pain.

During the practice of Zen, we learn all about pain. Zen meditation students sometimes sit for many hours on the cushion without moving. Sometimes there is incredible pain. As we continue to do this practice, we gradually become stronger than the pain and learn to see that all pain comes only from resistance, from fighting against the very moment. When we stop fighting, we experience joy. Once we start fighting again, we are cramped into agony.

> It was evening of the third day of retreat. We had been sitting (meditating) for seventeen hours a day. By now the pain was almost unbearable, and I was exhausted. I wanted to go home. I wanted my mother. I didn't know what I wanted. My legs were aching and my back was stiff. Now it was time for evening sitting. Three more hours to go. I didn't think I could make it.
>
> I sat down on my cushion and the bells rang out. After the bells, absolute silence. Soon the pain began to mount. There was no way at all I could escape it. The more I fought, the worse it became. Beside myself, I broke into the silence and started sobbing loudly. I knew I was disturbing everyone in the zendo but I couldn't help it. Still, the more I cried the worse I felt.
>
> Then, to my horror, Dogo, the head monk shouted out loudly at me, "Shut up or get out! Go sit by yourself down at the lake! Become stronger than the pain! There is no pain! You are the pain!"
>
> At that moment I let the struggle go. The pain went. I went. Instead there was incredible joy."
>
> Eshin

Being caught with a terminal illness and filled with pain is like being caught at a Zen retreat up in the mountains. No way out.

The way out is the way in.

Eido Roshi

The way out is to make friends with the pain.

Let us eliminate the doctor as well as the patient by accepting the disease itself.[2]

Henry Miller

Now, let us explore this attitude of *making friends* with the pain, with yourself, with your entire experience. What does this kind of attitude contain?

The attitude of *making friends* embodies the embracing of *all* our experience. We welcome everything, the good and the bad. We see it all as a way to grow, change, and develop. This kind of attitude is not interested in changing, using, or controlling a situation. It is mainly interested in exploring the situation (or person) and allowing it to be. This is a very gentle kind of attitude, an attitude of becoming acquainted.

During a time of illness and pain, we instinctively want to fight it off. We do not realize that fighting the pain intensifies it. Instead, we should welcome it, explore it, look at it kindly, many things will open up. There is a natural healing that is always available to us, but this energy is often cut off by tension and fear. When we let go and enter the flow of things, we become available to a greater source of help.

As soon as we feel pain, we usually tighten up. Our minds say that something terrible may be happening. But if we feel instead that something beautiful may be happening, we will not cramp up and clutch so. Sometimes it is not even the pain that is so terrible, but our thoughts and feelings about it, our fear that it signifies something awful.

[2]From *The Wisdom of the Heart,* by Henry Miller. Copyright 1941 by New Directions Publishing Corporation. Reprinted by permission of New Directions Publishing Corporation.

This kind of attitude can be applied not only to pain, but to all situations and all people. Let us learn more about the process of making friends.

Process

Who is your best friend? Why do you like your best friend so much? How do you feel when you are with your best friend? How are you with your best friend when you greet him or her? Try being that way with the pain too.

When we were children, it was easy to make friends. Now, as adults, we may have forgotten. The following process is to help us into that state of mind.

Process

Lie down on the floor. Take off your shoes; open your belt. (If there is a little cushion, put it under your head. If not, just lie there.)

Now, just feel whatever it is you are feeling. Let yourself gently become aware of whatever is going on inside of you, and around you. Take your time. Do not force your attention. Just let it go wherever it likes and follow it gently. How much space are you taking up? How does the air feel? Are you uncomfortable?

Don't try to get comfortable. What does it feel like to be uncomfortable? Sense it; let your body react to it in any way it might want to. Let your body find its own way to become comfortable. See if you can get out of the way.

Go ahead, make friends with your feelings, with whatever is there. Lie there and make friends with the floor. Let it support you. Let yourself enjoy it.

Exactly what does it mean for you to *make friends* with what is happening now? Feel this through as you are lying on the floor.

When you are ready, sit up slowly. Let yourself be aware of what it feels like to go from lying to sitting. Take a moment. Take another moment. All moments belong to you. Take them and feel them fully. These moments are who you are.

This attitude of making friends may be applied to anything that comes to you, including illness and pain. If you are ill, can you accept it, for the moment, find out about it, allow it in, and then allow it to go away? When you can do this, the illness is not something foreign and frightening, but just another part of your life.

In order to really make friends with our being, we must become aware, moment by moment, of what we are actually feeling, doing, and thinking about. In order to foster this kind of awareness, you must first be willing to say *yes* to whatever feelings come to you. Usually we push many feelings away, or judge them, or hate ourselves for having this or that particular one. We may also try to determine what we will feel and when we will feel it.

But, making friends means letting ourselves be and then discovering just who we are. It can become extremely shocking when we really begin to see ourselves. When feelings or responses emerge that we do not like, we can begin to hate ourselves for them. Most of us create impossible standards for how and who we should be. Then, when we do not live up to these fictitional standards, we suddenly fall into despair. This is not the attitude of making friends. This is the attitude of pain and constriction.

Making friends means welcoming all of your experiences; looking at them, knowing them and deeply accepting your humanity. This is the attitude of peace and healing. How accepting of yourself and others are you really? How much of a friend can you really be? The following process will explore these questions.

Process

To whom are you willing to be a real friend? Why? What about *that* person are you willing to accept? What about him or her do you find unacceptable?

What about yourself? What qualities are you willing to accept about yourself, to make friends with? What are the unacceptable parts and what do you do with them? Is what you do effective? Do the unacceptable parts ever go away?

Draw a picture of your unacceptable parts. Pretend to be one part; walk like it, talk like it. Now, as this unacceptable part, tell the rest of yourself what you think about it.

Look at the war caused by these unacceptable parts that is going on inside of you. Is reconciliation possible? Remember that conflict leads to illness and pain. What are you willing to do to help reconciliation?

Wellness is learning how to say *yes*. Wellness emerges out of the balance and harmony of all parts of ourselves. Wellness is the essence of reconciliation and does not come from fighting pain, but from acceptance and harmony.

When we are well, we are in harmony with ourselves and the world we live in. We cannot be in harmony with a mind that fights and rejects. Rejecting something never makes it go away, as it will come back over and over for us to reject again. Everything needs to be loved and accepted, including your illness and your pain.

Illness and pain may be thought to be expressions of our worst feelings, fears, and thoughts about ourselves. We must not shy away from them, but courageously face them, listen to them, and try to understand them.

Process

Look at your illness now. Do not run away from it. Just close your eyes and picture it within. Give it some kind of image or shape. What does it look like to you? Do you want to describe or draw it?

Now, look more deeply at what this image really means. What is this image saying to you about yourself and the life you are living? Let this image talk to you about yourself. What is it saying? Listen, just listen.

Next, ask it any questions you may have and let it answer you. If you would like to, ask this image exactly what it wants from you. Ask it what it would like in order for it to go away? Receive an answer.

Finally, picture yourself giving the image whatever it is asking for. Then picture it thanking you and going away.

This exercise may seem to be ridiculous to you, which is fine. In a sense it is ridiculous, but in another sense it is also valuable. This exercise puts us in touch with many of the feelings and thoughts that may not have been accessible to us before. This exercise is simply a way of learning how to talk to ourselves.

The judgment we often make that something is ridiculous, is simply a way of keeping ourselves from trying out something new. It is a way to keep ourselves in our old familiar patterns. So, accept your judgment that it is ridiculous, and then try it anyway.

This exercise comes out of a meditative approach to illness and pain. The *meditative attitude* does not view something objectively, from without, but enters into all experience. It becomes one with whatever it is applied to. This attitude wipes all distances and judgments away. The meditative attitude allows everything to be the teacher. In this vein, nothing then can be our enemy. If something is hurtful, it is still our teacher, and therefore ultimately our friend. This attitude does not intervene or interfere with experience, it simply allows our experience to speak for itself. It allows our life to be what it is. It allows the patient to know what he or she is needing. It is an attitude of great reverence and love.

Oddly enough, this attitude is not in conflict with medical treatment, because it is not in conflict with anything. When medical treatment is required, certainly it is offered, but it is offered with the meditative attitude. When we approach all situations with this kind of mind, alternate possibilities for helping become clear to us when they are needed.

This position holds a complete respect for each individual for his or her fundamental ability to know what is best for him or her. The role of the helper (family, friends, medical staff) here is not to control the patient, but to help the patient become in touch with what it is that he or she truly needs.

At times a patient may choose not to get well. The physician and family may take this as a personal injury. Each may feel like a failure.

We all have fixed notions about how patients *should* recover. We want them always to get well, strong, to make progress. But *progress* may look different for different people. Some truly need to go through a time of great disrepair. Part of the process of life includes times of illness and great pain. Out of the chaos and pain, more beauty and health can eventually appear. Sometimes we have to fall apart in order to be able to create ourselves anew.

Can you give the other person the right to have his or her own experience? Can you give this individual the right to make his or her own choices, not just for this illness, but for his or her whole life? Have you given yourself that right too?

Pain is mysterious. When we accept it and enter it, it disappears. Pain is only the lack of acceptance, the wish to be better than we feel we are. Each moment we live in acceptance, no matter how awful or strange the moment may be, this moment will not feel painful.

Pain is resistance against the flow. Resistance creates conflict and struggle. When there is no struggle, there is no pain and oneness comes, all by itself.

> *Imperceptibly*
> *The green leaves lengthen,*
> *Summer is near.*[3]
>
> Shiki

[3]From *Peonies Kana: Haiku by the Upasaka Shiki,* translated by Harold J. Isaacson. The Bhaisajaguru Series. Copyright © 1972 by Harold J. Isaacson. Used by permission of Theater Art Books, 153 Waverly Place, New York, NY 10014.

chapter ten
Being Born

The world is a womb, not a tomb, a place where everything is engendered and brought to life.[1]

Henry Miller

Just as we must learn how to die, we must also learn how to be born, to open our hearts, our minds, our eyes, and to grow constantly. To grow one inch is not enough.

Most of us live this incredible life half-dead and asleep, walking around in a dream. We are lost in sadness and in fear—a tremendous waste. Life is such a miraculous gift, which we refuse hour after hour, day after day. Why? Who are we to refuse this much beauty and joy?

We live on the edge of the miraculous every minute of our lives. The miracle is in us and it blossoms forth the moment we lay ourselves open to it. The miracle of miracles is the stubbornness with which we refuse to open ourselves up.[2]

Henry Miller

What must we do to really open up, to really become alive?

[1] From *The Wisdom of the Heart*, by Henry Miller. Copyright 1941 by New Directions Publishing Corporation. Reprinted by permission of New Directions Publishing Corporation.
[2] Miller, *The Wisdom of the Heart*.

First, we must learn to constantly throw everything we have to the winds, and let the wind bring back to us whatever it wants to, whenever it wants to. We limit ourselves because we are so busy holding on, with so many ideas of what we want from life. This very holding on keeps us from living and falling in love, over and over again.

To live fully requires courage and faith. We hear a great deal about the word *faith*, but what does it actually mean? Although there are many beliefs we carry, it is rare to really have faith in life itself and in our own life process. Instead, we feel bewildered by what is happening and try to stop and control it, to shape it to our particular wishes. Even though we may be very lost ourselves, we still want everything to go according to our own wishes.

When it does not, we become fearful and sad and do not know whose hand to hold. Then we begin to worry a lot about losing our direction. Day after day we can lose our direction.

But what is this precious direction that we want to hold onto so much? We may not yet have begun to see that all directions have the same destination, and that this destination is wonderful.

> *Walk to the left,*
> *Walk to the right,*
> *But above all,*
> *Don't fall down.*
>
> Old Zen saying

It's alright to fall down. You can just get up again. It can even be fun to lose your direction, but we are taught to be cautious and to hesitate. Yet the more we hesitate, the more we wobble and are afraid. In order to be truly alive, we must finally let go of this childish wobbling and all that it implies.

Many questions now arise:

How can I trust myself to know where to go; I am erratic.
How can I believe in myself?
How can I know that life is really good?

Faith implies taking a leap. It means being willing to stand up and walk bravely in spite of all that you do not know. It means trusting yourself even though you are erratic, accepting fundamentally that life is good, and believing life is wholesome and that you are always in good hands.

When you are good, life is good. When you are upset, life is terrifying. You may wonder, "So what if life is good? Why should I bother to live if someday I will have to die?" We resent old age and dying, but without dissolution of the old, nothing new can appear. All that is formed is subject to change. It cannot be any other way.

> *... form is no other than emptiness,*
> *Emptiness is no other than form;*
> *Form is exactly emptiness, emptiness exactly form,*
> *... all phenomena are emptiness/form ...*
>
> Heart Sutra

We must see that what we are is part of a formation, a coming together and falling away. Nothing is constant and everything is constant, and this exists simultaneously. Change itself is constant, and our particular lives change constantly.

> *I have always looked upon decay as being just as wonderful and rich an expression of life as growth.*[3]
>
> Henry Miller

Waste products become fertilizers for the soil much the way old ideas and ways become fertilizers for our new growth. It is all part of one circle. We must allow the old to dissolve in order to fertilize the new.

> *When alive, thoroughly alive,*
> *When dead, thoroughly dead.*
>
> Old Zen saying

Death is only another part of the cycle of our life. This is difficult for us to accept. We may want to protest and go on marches. But who are we to give orders? Why can't we allow the universe to be just the way it is? No one asked our opinion in the first place. If we do not interfere with the universe, then it will constantly replenish us, just

---

[3]Miller, *The Wisdom of the Heart.*

because it is its nature to do so. Look at the earth in spring and you will see.

> *The plum-tree of my hut;*
> *It couldn't be helped,*
> *It bloomed.*[4]

Shiki

We may not feel as if we deserve to live, to bloom, and to be constantly replenished. We have been taught to condemn and be ashamed of who we are. This deep self-condemnation will lead us to illness and death. This self-condemnation is itself the illness.

Process

Now, let us look at our own life process, at our own need to become born.

What does it mean to you to be really alive and well? Find a partner and share it with him or her. Share your ideas any way you like; by drawing, singing, talking, dancing.

For this next process, there are two partners. The first person says the sentence aloud and completes it spontaneously. Each sentence is done several times. The second person listens and simply says, "thank you." When each partner is finished, reverse roles.

To be really alive is _____.
The part of me that is really alive is _____.
The part of me that is most dead is _____.
The part of me that wants to get born is _____.

What part of you has to die in order for another part to get born? Are you willing to let it die?

We must learn to make friends with all the parts of ourselves, the parts we want to keep and the parts we want to let go. Most of us think we are stuck with ourselves and have to be this way forever.

[4]From *Peonies Kana: Haiku by the Upasaka Shiki*, translated by Harold J. Isaacson. The Bhaisajaguru Series. Copyright © 1972 by Harold J. Isaacson. Used by permission of Theater Art Books, 153 Waverly Place, New York, NY 10014.

Others feel they have to die in order to start all over again. Others may go and hide up in the mountains.

But, you can start all over again right now. It is really very simple because there are endless possibilities within you. You just have to be willing to allow them to appear. It's like having a room and changing the furniture. First spring cleaning, then getting new furniture and new colors, change a little bit at a time.

Process

This is a guided meditation that will help you see the parts of yourself that want to be born and the parts that are ready to go away. You will need a friend to read the instructions slowly and gently. This process may be done in a group, or just with two people. Some enjoy hearing soft music in the background while it is going on.

Close your eyes, relax, and become at ease. Now, picture yourself in a place you love to be, a place you feel safe and happy. Look at the place closely; how do you feel now? If you like, you may picture a nearby road.

Now, get an image of the part of yourself that would like to be born. (If you like, you may personify the part and visualize the part coming along down the road.) What is he or she like? Look at him or her closely. Make friends with him or her. Does he or she have a name? Where does he or she live? What does he or she like to do? What kind of songs does he or she like to sing? Is there something he or she wants to say to you? Is there something you may wish to reply? Is there some particular person or friend he or she wants nearby?

Now, ask yourself, what is in the way of this person being born? Get another image, as an answer to the question. See what this image means; look closely at the difficulty. Talk to it. Let it reply. Ask it, what is it doing there in the way? What does it want? What is it afraid of? What is required in order for the obstacle to go away? See if you can give it to him or her. Be very gentle with yourself. You are not going to obliterate the obstacle, you are simply going to let it go away.

When you are ready, open your eyes and come back to the room. Now, get some crayons and draw a picture as the "new person" you found would draw it. Have this new person introduce him- or herself to the others. Let the person tell his or her name, or sing a song, or give a gift, or ask for a gift. Let the new person do whatever he or she may like. Do not be afraid to use your imagination. Really feel what it feels like to be this new person. Can you allow him or her to just be there and to live?

This process is extremely enjoyable and illuminating for many. It can quickly bring us in touch with the endless possibilities that always exist within us for new experience, new expression, and new adventure.

When we really see that we are presently alive, and always in the process of becoming, we see that we never have to grow stale and dead. Dying may be here just to remind us that it is time to get born again. Until we are born we are only seedlings.

A book about death inevitably has to be a book about birth also. Death and birth are times when we come to know who we truly are, and what is really possible for us. These are times when we can come to our peak experiences, to the fullness of knowing ourselves. These points are also times when many people begin to come to prayer.

It is impossible to write a book on dying without talking about prayer. Very few of us really know what prayer is, or dream of taking it seriously. For many, a prayer is simply a repetition of old, childlike behavior, mainly inspired by fear. Actually, prayer is the fulfillment of man's development. It is an activity through which man grows into as his childishness falls away.

We have become extremely confused about this matter. In our society and training, prayer is considered superstitious and irrational. We do it (when we do it) out of rote and out of respect for "tradition." But, most of us have no idea at all of what constitutes true prayer. Even though we attend a thousand church or temple services, we may still not have tasted true prayer.

Prayer is the very door to our center. It is the key that unlocks our heart and our larger understanding. Prayer is an activity, a way of being in the world. It is the very process of becoming one with all beings and of regarding them with reverence and awe. Most of us think that prayer is "asking for something." This is not necessarily prayer.

Commonly prayers are offered for long life, health, wealth, happiness, and so on. This is a childlike kind of prayer where we ask to be given to. It comes from feeling needful and empty. It is not an overflowing, an offering, which comes from feeling full. There is nothing wrong with this kind of prayer, but it is just merely the very beginning. It is an initial impulse to walk along this path of understanding.

Some offer prayers for repentence, arising out of deep feelings of guilt. These are the prayers that are asking that we be cleansed of our sins. Some feel better after these kinds of prayers, some feel much worse. Embedded deep within this kind of praying is the notion that we are sinful and bad.

Some may refuse to pray because they have no idea of who they are praying to. "I feel foolish. I don't know if there is anyone there. I don't really think anyone will answer me."

Prayer is its own answer. Inevitably an answer will come, one way or another. Probably it will not be the answer you were expecting, and certainly not in the way you imagined. To really pray deeply, you must let go of all your preconceived expectations and just pray.

Prayer is a natural human function that has been severely repressed and distorted for many. Prayer has a natural healing power. It has an expanding, soothing, clarifying effect. Just as it is natural for the human being to seek friendship, it is natural for a human to turn toward prayer. During a time of illness and dying, it is extremely beneficial to turn toward prayer. What does it mean to pray deeply and truly? What is prayer exactly? How may you experience it?

A state of prayer is a state of mind, a way of being in the world. Prayer itself has different forms, but these forms only exist in order to bring us to that state of mind.

To pray means to turn toward our larger being, to our greater selves, and to establish communication. We can make an offering. Some feel that to pray is to give a gift. In the state of prayer, we are relating ourselves to something larger than our own personal selves. We may be inviting this larger sense of life to permeate our entire being, and our relations with others.

For some prayer means chanting, for others singing, meditating, dancing, bowing, or working with love in their own garden. The mind of prayer is a mind that is giving thanks for the gift of life and is willing to celebrate life continually. It is a state of mind that beautifies its surroundings.

Bowing is a very serious practice. You should be prepared to bow, even in your last moment. Even though it is impossible to get rid of our self-centered desires, we have to do it. Our true nature wants us to.[5]

Suzuki Roshi

Prayer is a way of listening to and discovering our true nature, and of living with it daily. This true nature is with us constantly, before we were born and after we die. It can make us very happy, if we allow it to.

Prayer becomes very, very necessary because it is easy to forget. Many of us become like ungrateful guests at the marvellous banquet of life. We are the guests who are upset that the meal will not last forever. We criticize the food we are receiving. We want this food and we do not like that. We gorge ourselves greedily, fearing that there will never be enough. Then, there is always something unpleasant we have to say about all the other guests. We have no idea at all who our host is, or why we have been invited here. We focus only upon the food on the table, and never dream of offering thanks.

Some don't care what they are doing here, they only want to eat. When the food runs out, they simply feel terrified. Others don't care so much about the food, they just want to push everyone else around. They are under the illusion that this is their party. They do not realize that they are just more guests, along with the birds and the bees that appear here. They are not willing to admit that all deserve to eat at the same table.

Some refuse to eat the meal entirely and go pout in the corner, waiting for the party to end.

Prayer is a way of looking for the host, offering thanks, and maybe of beginning to discover just why we have been invited here. Prayer says, "thank you," eats its fill, and then asks, "what can I offer in return?" As we pray we begin to see that each person is here at this banquet for a reason. There is something they particularly have to add. It is quite an adventure to discover what *you* have to offer to this party.

When we are dying and in agony, it may be difficult to turn our minds toward prayer for the first time. When prayer is included in our daily life, however, it becomes a through-line that is taken with

[5]From *Zen Mind, Beginner's Mind,* by Suzuki Roshi, Weatherhill, 1970.

us. Prayer is simply a way of remembering that we have not always been here and that one day we will be departing. It helps us to be conscious and loving of the others in this world.

There are many different ways or praying, and of attaining and maintaining this state of mind. We do not have to pray only at designated times and places (although this may be very helpful to some).

Work may become a form of prayer as well, when it is done in this state of mindfulness. A physician with a patient and a carpenter with wood, may both be engaged in the activity of praying.

Bowing deeply (within or without) to one another, and letting go of our self-centered opinions and demanding ways, is a fine kind of praying.

Process

Look at your child (or friend, lover, whomever), and bow to him or her first thing in the morning.

Bow to this person before you offer him or her food. See how you feel after you do this. (If you are too embarrassed to do this so he can see it, do it in your mind. Stop for a moment, pause, and make a bow to whomever you are in an interaction with. You are bowing out of respect and reverence for his or her life and yours.)

As we pray deeply, we gradually become empty and clean. We become one with the entire universe and lose our sense of alienation. This is an invocation of the highest and the best we are capable of.

Prayer is an act of deep surrender. It is a way of saying *yes* to our existence and to one another. We are letting go of the notion that we are so special, better than the other, and that the entire world revolves around us. We are allowing ourselves to be instructed and to be guided. We are allowing the other to become our teacher, our partner, and our true friend.

A life and practice of continuing prayer is the best possible preparation to greet our dying, and our birthing. It is the best possible instruction to live most fully, with the greatest understanding.

All that we are, that we need, and that we know is already deep within. True prayer opens this house of treasure for us.

Appendix

Following are alternative ways of growth, opening, and enhanced understanding that are particularly useful during the time of death and parting.

Alexander Technique
Rupa Cousins
   (certified practitioner)
415 Central Park West
New York, NY 10025
(212) 662-6699

   This practice deals with the body and with gentle touching, which helps to release memories and unblock the energy flow.

DiMele Center for
   Psychotherapy
Armand DiMele
15 East 40 Street
New York, NY 10016
(212) 889-5555

   This practice deals with the intense feeling process. It allows us to express and experience deep emotions and memories. This is particularly useful during a time of grief.

Health Support Group
Mr. Gene Pometto,
Dr. Robert Atkins
4505 Elsrode Avenue
Baltimore, MD 21214

The purpose of this group is to assist and support people who are experiencing difficult life changes. The services include group therapeutic and health promoting techniques. Both mental and physical health and its co-relationship is handled. Issues addressed include the interdependent relationship between physical and mental health, barriers to positive lifestyle changes, coping with stress, nutrition and diet, meditation and yoga, and cardiovascular conditioning.

Huna
Norman Francini
1365 York Avenue
New York, NY 10021
(212) 737-9182

This is beautiful, gentle work from the ancient teachings of Hawaii. In a loving and playful manner, it helps us to transform pain and negativity into light, love, and growth.

Loving Relationships
   Training
Sondra Ray (creator)
Charlotte Weiser
   (organizer)
433 W. 34th Street
New York, NY 10001
(212) 564-8502

This is a weekend training designed to examine our relationships and see what prevents us from giving and receiving love. It is intended to open our ability to love others and ourselves.

Rebirthing
Robert Mandel
    (certified practitioner)
Mallie Burzon
    (certified practitioner)
145 West 87 Street
New York, NY 10024
(212) 799-7323

Theta San Francisco
Lenord Orr
545 11th Avenue
San Francisco, CA 94118
(415) 221-2868

Campbell Hot Springs
P.O. Box 38
Sierraville, CA 96126
(916) 994-8894

Michael Green
40 Longfellow St.
Dorchester, MA
(617) 265-0755

Rebirth International
Rima Beth Star
P.O. Box 10205
Austin, Texas 78757
(512) 453-8194

This is a breathing therapy created by Lenord Orr that is designed to take us back to the time of our birth and help us release all the trauma and negative thoughts we created then. The result of this is to help us live in the present and feel safe, loved, and positive, enjoying and caring for our bodies.

Sedona Institute
Lester Levenson
30 East 76th Street
New York, NY 10021
(212) 861-2380

Sedona Institute
Dr. Robert Scott
Star Route, Box 264
Sausalito, CA 94965
(415) 383-3150)

Sedona Institute
2408 Arizona Biltmore
    Circle
Phoenix, AZ 85016
(602) 956-8765

This is a gentle, clear, two weekend course which provides a simple and powerful tool which helps to release stress. This tool teaches us how to "let go" of negativity so that we can experience freedom and fullness regardless of the external circumstances we find ourselves in.

The Practice of Zazen;
Zen meditation

New York Area:

Chan Medical Center
90-31 Corona Avenue
Queens, NY
(212) 592-6593

The New York Zendo
Eido Roshi
223 East 67 Street
New York, NY 10021
(212) 861-3333

The First Zen Institute
Sassaki Roshi
113 East 30 Street
New York, NY 10016
(212) MU4-9487

Zen Community of New
   York
Glassman Sensei
Greystone Avenue
Riverdale, NY 10471
(212) 543-5530

Additional Centers for Zen Meditation:

Zen Center of Los Angeles
Maezumi Roshi
927 S. Normandie Avenue
Los Angeles, CA 90006
(213) 387-2351

Mt. Baldy Zen Center
Joshu Sassaki Roshi
Mt. Baldy, CA 91759-0429
(714) 865-6410

Zen Center
300 Page Street
San Francisco, CA 94102
(415) 863-3136

Cimarron Zen Center
Sassaki Roshi
2505 Cimarron Street
Los Angeles, CA 90018
(213) 732-2263

Cambridge Zen Center
Seung Sahn Soen-sa
Cambridge, MA
(617) 254-0363

The Providence Zen Center
Seung Sahn Soen-sa
R.F.D. 5
Pound Road
Cumberland, RI 02864
(401) 769-6464

Jemez Bodhi Mandala
Sassaki Roshi
Box 44
Jemez Springs, NM 97025

Zazen is the practice of Zen meditation; sitting quietly and walking mindfully. It helps clear our minds and lives of stray thoughts and desires so that we can live simply and lucidly.

Sitting quietly and doing nothing,
spring comes
and the grass grows by itself.

GROUPS THAT WORK DIRECTLY WITH
THE SERIOUSLY ILL AND THEIR FAMILIES

Center for Attitudinal Healing
Dr. Gerald G. Jampolsky
19 Main Street
Tiburon, CA 94920
(415) 435-5022
(Specializing in children.)

Attitudinal Healing Center
of Long Island
1691 Northern Blvd.
Manhasset, NY 11021
(516) 869-8118

Richard Boerstler
206 Maplewood Street
Watertown, MA 02172
(617) 923-9278

Eve Boden, C.S.W.
175 Jericho Turnpike
Suite 316
Syosset, NY 11791
(516) 496-8222

Hanuman Foundation
Ram Dass
2043 Francisco Street
Berkeley, CA 94709

Hospice, Inc.
765 Prospect St.
New Haven, Conn. 06511
(203) 787-5871
(Center of national network
of hospices.)

Hospice of Bloomington
Gwen Galsworth
316 North Washington St.
Bloomington, IN 47401
(812) 339-5177

Association for Humanistic Psychology

Association for
  Humanistic Psychology
325 Ninth Street
San Francisco, CA 94103
(415) 626-2375)

Association for
  Humanistic Psychology
Midwest Regional Office
7011 North Greenview
Chicago, IL 60626
(312) 465-7367

Association for
  Humanistic Psychology
Tucker Ranson,
Puja Tobey
Eastern Regional Office
2 Washington Square Village
New York, NY 10012
(212) 674-8785

This organization provides on-going conferences, both regionally and nationally in which a wide variety of workshops are offered which deal with many new aspects of health care. Also offered are workshops dealing with lifestyle, value clarification, and general wellness.

Interface
Dr. Rick Ingrasci
63 Chapel Street
Newton, MA 02158
(617) 964-7140
    A center providing workshops and courses related to all matters and alternative health care and holistic health.

Network for Life Changes
Ian Raffel
Vancouver, V6 02
British Col.
(604) 738-8466
    These are stress management consultants dealing in corrective body work, alternative health care practices.

SAGE (Senior Actuali-
zation and Growth
Exploration)
P.O. Box 4244
San Francisco, CA 04101
(415) 763-0965
   Workshops and material dedicated to creating and imple-
menting a new image regarding aging; one filled with life, vitality and
growth.

Shanti Project
Dr. Kübler-Ross
1137 Colusa Street
Berkeley, CA 94909
(415) 524-4370

Shell of Hope
2584 National Drive
Brooklyn, NY 11234
(212) 763-0827

Waterfarm
Ben Hopkins
RR 3 Box 206
Chestertown, MD 21620
   A unique community designed for living and practicing in a
loving, clear manner. Here there is an attempt to combine heart and
mind, values and technology for the enrichment of life in society.

Bibliography

Following is a list of books referred to in the text.
BUBER, MARTIN, *Tales of the Hasidim.* New York: Schocken Books, 1966.
——, *Between Man and Man.* New York: Schocken Books, 1965.
CAMUS, ALBERT, *The Stranger.* New York: Vintage Press, 1946.
MILLER, HENRY, *The Wisdom of the Heart.* New York: New Directions, 1960.
ORR, LENARD, *Rebirthing in the New Age.* Millbrae, Calf.: Celestial Arts, 1977.
RAJNEESH, BHAGWAN SHREE, *Zen: Zest, Zip, Zap, and Zing.* Poona, India: Rajneesh Foundation, 1981.
ROSHI, EIDO, SENZAKI ROSHI, and SOEN ROSHI, *Namu Dai Bosa.* The Bhaisajaguru Series, New York: Theater Arts Books, 1976.
SHIKI, *Peonies Kana.* The Bhaisajaguru Series, New York: Theater Arts Books, 1972.
SUZUKI, ROSHI, *Zen Mind, Beginner's Mind.* New York: Weatherhill, 1970.

Following is a list of recommended supplementary readings.
DAVIS, BRUCE, *The Magical Child Within You.* Millbrae, Calf.: Celestial Arts, 1977.
EMERSON, RALPH WALDO, *Self Reliance.* New York: Funk and Wagnalls, 1975.

KAPLEAU, PHILIP, *The Three Pillars of Zen.* New York: Beacon, 1965.

PRATHER, HUGH, *Notes to Myself.* Moab: Real Peoples Press, 1970.

TRUNGPA, CHOGYAM, *The Tibetan Book of the Dead.* Berkley, Calf. Shambhala, 1975.

———, *Meditation in Action.* Berkley, Calf.: Shambhala, 1969.

WATTS, ALAN W., *The Wisdom of Insecurity.* New York: Vintage, 1951.

WHITMAN, WALT, *Leaves of Grass.* New York: Mentor, 1954.

Index